Beyond Lip Service

This book underscores the importance of moving beyond lip service or hollow platitudes to mobilize and expand the capacity of social justice movements to foster policy change and incubate new programs at the local, state, and federal levels.

In the wake of global protests spurred by acts of police brutality in the United States, the present-day problematic policing and racial injustice in Black and Brown communities surged to the forefront of political discourse in recent years. Institutionalized backlash politics, which emerged during the post-Civil Rights era, perpetuated and further exacerbated generations-long racial disparities and stymied systemic change. This edited volume describes pilot programs and community-based initiatives that show promise as tools for equity and racial justice in Black and Brown communities.

This book will be of great value to scholars and academics interested in racism, justice, community development, and social work. The chapters in this book were originally published in the *Journal of Community Practice*.

Anna Maria Santiago is Professor in the College of Social Science at Michigan State University, East Lansing, USA. Her research focuses on community development and the geography of opportunity, financial capability and asset building, and neighborhood effects on child health and well-being in Latinx, African American, and immigrant communities.

Kelly Patterson is Associate Professor in the School of Social Work at the University at Buffalo, USA. Her research focuses on subsidized housing, racial segregation, fair housing advocacy, social policy, and social service access/delivery.

Robert Mark Silverman is Professor in the Department of Urban and Regional Planning at the University at Buffalo, USA. His research focuses on community development, community-based organizations, education reform, and inequality in inner-city housing markets.

Beyond Lip Service

Bringing Racial Justice to Black and Brown Communities

Edited by
Anna Maria Santiago, Kelly Patterson
and Robert Mark Silverman

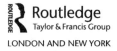

LONDON AND NEW YORK

First published 2023
by Routledge
4 Park Square, Milton Park, Abingdon, Oxon, OX14 4RN

and by Routledge
605 Third Avenue, New York, NY 10158

Routledge is an imprint of the Taylor & Francis Group, an informa business

Chapters 1–8 © 2023 Taylor & Francis

All rights reserved. No part of this book may be reprinted or reproduced or utilised in any form or by any electronic, mechanical, or other means, now known or hereafter invented, including photocopying and recording, or in any information storage or retrieval system, without permission in writing from the publishers.

Trademark notice: Product or corporate names may be trademarks or registered trademarks, and are used only for identification and explanation without intent to infringe.

British Library Cataloguing-in-Publication Data
A catalogue record for this book is available from the British Library

ISBN13: 978-1-032-41540-6 (hbk)
ISBN13: 978-1-032-41542-0 (pbk)
ISBN13: 978-1-003-35861-9 (ebk)

DOI: 10.4324/9781003358619

Typeset in Minion Pro
by codeMantra

Publisher's Note
The publisher accepts responsibility for any inconsistencies that may have arisen during the conversion of this book from journal articles to book chapters, namely the inclusion of journal terminology.

Disclaimer
Every effort has been made to contact copyright holders for their permission to reprint material in this book. The publishers would be grateful to hear from any copyright holder who is not here acknowledged and will undertake to rectify any errors or omissions in future editions of this book.

Contents

	Citation Information	vi
	Notes on Contributors	viii
1	The enduring backlash against racial justice in the United States: mobilizing strategies for institutional change *Kelly Patterson, Anna Maria Santiago, and Robert Mark Silverman*	1
2	Removing the knees from their necks: mobilizing community practice and social action for racial justice *Anna Maria Santiago and Jan Ivery*	12
3	From the archives: the Los Angeles riot study *Paul H. Stuart*	25
4	Beyond community policing: centering community development in efforts to improve safety in Latinx immigrant communities *Willow Lung-Amam, Nohely Alvarez, and Rodney Green*	42
5	Bursting bubbles: outcomes of an intergroup contact intervention within the context of a community based violence intervention program *Christopher St. Vil and Kwasi Boaitey*	58
6	Can preference policies advance racial justice? *Amie Thurber, Lisa K. Bates, and Susan Halverson*	72
7	Minority Political Leadership Institute: a model for developing racial equity leadership *Nakeina E. Douglas-Glenn, Shabana K. Shaheen,* *Elizabeth P. Marlowe, and Kiara S. Faulks*	90
8	Toward authentic university-community engagement *Mark G. Chupp, Adrianne M. Fletcher, and James P. Graulty*	102
	Index	117

Citation Information

The chapters in this book, except for chapter 2, were originally published in the *Journal of Community Practice*, volume 29, issue 4 (2021). Chapter 2 was originally published in volume 28, issue 3 (2020) of the same journal. When citing this material, please use the original page numbering for each article, as follows:

Chapter 1
The enduring backlash against racial justice in the United States: mobilizing strategies for institutional change
Kelly Patterson, Anna Maria Santiago, and Robert Mark Silverman
Journal of Community Practice, volume 29, issue 4 (2021) pp. 334–344

Chapter 2
Removing the knees from their necks: mobilizing community practice and social action for racial justice
Anna Maria Santiago and Jan Ivery
Journal of Community Practice, volume 28, issue 3 (2020) pp. 195–207

Chapter 3
From the archives: the Los Angeles riot study
Paul H. Stuart
Journal of Community Practice, volume 29, issue 4 (2021) pp. 345–361

Chapter 4
Beyond community policing: centering community development in efforts to improve safety in Latinx immigrant communities
Willow Lung-Amam, Nohely Alvarez, and Rodney Green
Journal of Community Practice, volume 29, issue 4 (2021) pp. 375–390

Chapter 5
Bursting bubbles: outcomes of an intergroup contact intervention within the context of a community based violence intervention program
Christopher St. Vil and Kwasi Boaitey
Journal of Community Practice, volume 29, issue 4 (2021) pp. 391–404

Chapter 6

Can preference policies advance racial justice?
Amie Thurber, Lisa K. Bates, and Susan Halverson
Journal of Community Practice, volume 29, issue 4 (2021) pp. 405–422

Chapter 7

Minority Political Leadership Institute: a model for developing racial equity leadership
Nakeina E. Douglas-Glenn, Shabana K. Shaheen, Elizabeth P. Marlowe, and Kiara S. Faulks
Journal of Community Practice, volume 29, issue 4 (2021) pp. 423–434

Chapter 8

Toward authentic university-community engagement
Mark G. Chupp, Adrianne M. Fletcher, and James P. Graulty
Journal of Community Practice, volume 29, issue 4 (2021) pp. 435–449

For any permission-related enquiries please visit:
http://www.tandfonline.com/page/help/permissions

Notes on Contributors

Nohely Alvarez, School of Architecture, Planning and Preservation, University of Maryland, College Park, USA.

Lisa K. Bates, Toulan School of Urban Studies and Planning, Portland State University, USA.

Kwasi Boaitey, Department of Health Humanities and Bioethics, University of Rochester, USA.

Mark G. Chupp, Jack, Joseph and Morton Mandel School of Applied Social Sciences, Case Western Reserve University, Cleveland, USA.

Nakeina E. Douglas-Glenn, L. Douglas Wilder School of Government and Public Affairs, Virginia Commonwealth University, Richmond, USA.

Kiara S. Faulks, L. Douglas Wilder School of Government and Public Affairs, Virginia Commonwealth University, Richmond, USA.

Adrianne M. Fletcher, Jack, Joseph and Morton Mandel School of Applied Social Sciences, Case Western Reserve University, Cleveland, USA.

James P. Graulty, Jack, Joseph and Morton Mandel School of Applied Social Sciences, Case Western Reserve University, Cleveland, USA.

Rodney Green, Center for Urban Progress, Howard University, Washington DC, USA.

Susan Halverson, School of Social Work, Portland State University, USA.

Jan Ivery, School of Social Work, Georgia State University, Atlanta, USA.

Willow Lung-Amam, School of Architecture, Planning and Preservation, University of Maryland, College Park, USA.

Elizabeth P. Marlowe, L. Douglas Wilder School of Government and Public Affairs, Virginia Commonwealth University, Richmond, USA.

Kelly Patterson, School of Social Work, University at Buffalo, USA.

Anna Maria Santiago, College of Social Science, Michigan State University, East Lansing, USA.

Shabana K. Shaheen, L. Douglas Wilder School of Government and Public Affairs, Virginia Commonwealth University, Richmond, USA.

Robert Mark Silverman, Department of Urban and Regional Planning, University at Buffalo, USA.

NOTES ON CONTRIBUTORS

Paul H. Stuart, School of Social Work, Florida International University, USA.

Christopher St. Vil, School of Social Work, University at Buffalo, USA.

Amie Thurber, School of Social Work, Portland State University, USA.

The enduring backlash against racial justice in the United States: mobilizing strategies for institutional change

Kelly Patterson, Anna Maria Santiago, and Robert Mark Silverman ⓘ

Introduction

This essay offers a framework for contextualizing racial injustice in contemporary Black and Brown communities. We argue that present-day racial injustice in the United States is a continuation of historical patterns of discrimination that have been institutionalized and reaffirmed for centuries (Gordon-Reed, 2021). At the same time, we underscore how racism and racial injustice have assumed distinctive forms during the post-civil rights era. While the passage of civil rights legislation in the 1960s represented a watershed moment in our history, it also triggered sustained backlash from opponents to racial justice in the United States (Glickman, 2020). This legislation and opposition during the post-civil rights era is significant because of the scope and magnitude of the policies adopted, as well as resistance to them. Legislation such as the 1964 Civil Rights Act, the 1964 Economic Opportunity Act, the 1965 Voting Rights Act, the 1965 Immigration and Naturalization Act, and the 1968 Fair Housing Act have been flashpoints for resistance (Boussac, 2021; Rieder, 1989). From its inception, opponents worked feverishly to dismantle these legislative acts which were encapsulated under the umbrella of the War on Poverty. Largely, their efforts have resulted in the curtailment and reversal of civil rights policies. It is notable that this opposition was built on a foundation of sustained discourse drawing from right-wing ideologies supporting racism and oppression, racial microaggressions, stereotypes and tropes mobilized to block the implementation of civil rights policies, and reconstructed color lines in the United States (Boussac, 2021; Rieder, 1989).

We offer this framework as a reference point for contextualizing the articles in this special issue on racial justice in Black and Brown communities. As the title of the special issue suggests, this framework is introduced in order to move beyond paying lip service to the topics covered in these articles. Understanding how racial discourse has been used (and misused) by opponents of civil rights is critical. We argue that opposition to civil rights legislation emerged as an organizing principle of the political right in the United States during the early 1960s. Although overlooked, this shift in political strategy is arguably one of the more successful policy agendas implemented during the contemporary period. Political conservatives, who constitute the right-wing in the United States, framed civil rights policies as failures from their inception, starved them of necessary fiscal resources, lobbied to reverse them, and defined social justice movements as undemocratic, unfair, and a subterfuge for patronage politics and clientelism.

In the section that follows, we discuss how backlash to racial justice policies has been institutionalized in the United States. As we witness continued calls for social workers to collaborate with police in order to reduce racist incidents and help improve the tenuous relationships between law enforcement and Black and Brown communities, the profession also is being challenged to examine the ways in which it has been and continues to be complicit in perpetuating racial injustice (see Santiago & Ivery, 2020). As the profession seemingly pays lip service to ending structural and systemic discrimination in housing, schools, workplaces, neighborhoods, and communities, we propose strategies for social workers, community practitioners, advocates, and activists to more effectively mobilize, respond to, and dismantle institutional racism.

Institutionalized backlash politics

The silent majority is a backstop against civil rights

The post-civil rights era has been shaped by an organized effort on the political right to dismantle federal legislation passed during the War on Poverty. During this period, the right-wing began to implement their *southern strategy* to galvanize their core populist constituency – a constituency that was re-branded as the *silent majority* to serve as a backstop against civil rights (Piven & Cloward, 1971; Rieder, 1989). Achieving Republican electoral victories by stoking racial animus among disaffected whites was the end goal. The southern strategy was central to Barry Goldwater's failed attempt to win the presidency in 1964 and Richard Nixon's successful effort to win the White House in 1968. A core component of the southern strategy was to galvanize racial resentment, oppose civil rights legislation, and cultivate anti-government sentiment among white voters. This strategy was used to rouse the silent majority (i.e., disaffected white voters) and foment a sustained backlash aimed at blocking the implementation of civil rights legislation and ultimately dismantling it. The southern strategy was distinct for two reasons. First, it represented an open effort to institutionalize an anti-civil rights agenda based on racial grievances in right-wing politics. Second, it was nurtured since the early 1960s to form a sustained effort at local, state, and national levels to systematically challenge and dismantle civil rights legislation (Glickman, 2020).

In its most visceral expression, the southern strategy was used to promote the right wing populist movement's focus on "a recurring rhetoric that vowed to protect white, middle-class taxpayers from the governing elite who allegedly wasted people's money on undeserving minorities" (Boussac, 2021, p. 183).

This rhetoric was successfully mobilized to differing degrees by other national politicians including George Wallace, Ronald Reagan, George H.W. Bush, George W. Bush, and Donald Trump. It also has been reinforced at the state and local levels as a sustained narrative to reverse civil rights and preserve the status quo. In total, the southern strategy has been the bedrock of the anti-civil rights agenda for over a half century.

A distinguishing characteristic of the right-wing populist movement is that its attack on the welfare state is based on a rhetorical web of stereotypes and racial tropes that provide the pretense for the use of microaggressions and more subtle forms of racist behaviors. These talking points are then deployed in an organized fashion to reinforce a belief system that buffers the status quo against efforts to promote institutional reform and critique racism (Santiago & Ivery, 2020). This discourse has taken different forms over the decades. In the 1960s and 1970s, social welfare policies were attacked as conduits for the promotion of a culture of poverty that spread social pathologies intergenerationally in the country's inner cities (Santiago, 2015). Leading into the 1980s, this discourse evolved and took on new dimensions. Attacks intensified, with opponents arguing that social welfare policies resulted in the disintegration of the nuclear family. One iconic right-wing attack deployed by Ronald Reagan and others during this period argued that the social safety net rewarded Black, "'welfare queens' who drove Cadillacs while claiming benefits" (Boussac, 2021, p. 197). The image of the welfare queen became embedded in subsequent scholarly debate about the underclass and the undeserving poor (Katz, 1990; Levine, 2018; Murray, 1985; Peterson & Rom, 1990; Wilson, 1990).

The right-wing movement's rhetorical attacks were not confined to the welfare state. They were applied across a spectrum of civil rights reforms. For example, the mobilization of white animus has been a central component of the campaign against immigration reform (Brown, 2013; Zolberg, 1999). White animus also has been mobilized in efforts to dismantle the Voting Rights Act of 1965 (Feagin & Hohle, 2017). Racism was a subtext of policy debates about healthcare in the 1990s (Boychuk, 2008) and early 2000s (Maxwell & Shields, 2014; Milner & Franz, 2020). Stereotypes were mobilized to thwart efforts to expand fair and affordable housing programs (Silverman & Patterson, 2012; Silverman et al., 2021). Similarly, efforts to promote criminal justice reform were repeatedly thwarted through references to racialized stereotypes and appeals to white fear (Lane et al., 2020; Owens, 2020).

Squashing the fruits of black political gains and social justice movements

The existence of an institutionalized backlash to civil rights has undermined political gains made in Black, Brown and other minoritized communities. This has been the case both in terms of gains made when minorities win elected offices and grassroots movements anchored in civil disobedience and civil unrest. Electoral gains by minority candidates have been described as a *hollow prize*, particularly when they are made in local elections (Friesema, 1969; Kraus & Swanstrom, 2001; Reed, 1988). When minorities win mayoral elections, they often inherit cities that have experienced disinvestment and population decline. The cities they govern are stigmatized by the broader society through the mobilization of stereotypes and tropes that are core components of the right-wing backlash to the civil rights movement. Minority-led cities are characterized as places where intergenerational poverty is sustained by welfare dependence, public corruption, and failed social policies. This type of framing places constraints on the scope of local redistributive policies that minority mayors can pursue. In order to placate the local and regional business interests, minority mayors face pressure to abandon redistributive agendas focused on making investments in social infrastructure, and instead they focus on things like business retention and the policing of the residential population (Bennett, 1993; Johnson, 2016; Reed, 1988). Ironically, they abandon the agendas of the local coalitions that brought them into power in order to show a response to right-wing political rhetoric that is deployed to dismantle civil rights policies.

The notion of a hollow prize has application at the state and federal levels of government as well. Black and Brown elected officials and their allies face obstacles to achieving legislative goals that are both an outgrowth of opposition driven by right-wing backlash and consequently embedded in institutional structures (Sekou, 2020). In the contemporary period, this is exemplified by stalled legislation at the federal level related to criminal justice reform, immigration reform, healthcare policy, fair housing, voting rights, and other civil rights issues. In the same way the reform agendas of Black and Brown mayors are blocked by the threat of accelerated disinvestment, efforts to implement civil rights and social justice reforms are blocked at the state and federal levels by backlash politics designed to maintain the status quo.

It is important to highlight that backlash is used to generate conflict, reframe political discourse, and disrupt democratic processes. It has emerged during the past half century in response to repeated cycles of civil disobedience aimed at addressing civil rights violations and social injustice. During the 1960s and early-1970s, backlash surfaced in response to the civil rights movement. As Black-led protests were gaining support from the public and through legislative initiative, opponents to civil rights reform encourage backlash and reframed protest movements as violent (Wasow, 2020). The reframing of social justice movements as violent led to waning public support for civil rights reforms. Similarly, after the 1992 acquittal of police officers videotaped beating Rodney King in Los Angeles and the civil unrest and disorder that ensued, there was increased support at the local level for policy reforms aimed at addressing the underlying structural inequalities that produced these mass acts of civil disobedience (Enos et al., 2019). Yet, local policy reforms did not translate into change at the national level. Instead, reframing of the Los Angeles civil uprisings as opportunistic rioting detached from the root causes of civil disobedience produced a backlash that effectively blocked efforts for changes in national policy. The ongoing inability of social justice movements to produce tangible policy change at the national level continues to be identified as a point of concern. For instance, Szetela (2020, p. 1367) argues that the ability of the Black Lives Matter movement to have a legislative impact at the state and federal levels is dubious, in part, because the "conservative backlash would have unprecedented ammunition for its race-charged destruction of the social welfare state."

From shock troops to institutional barriers to social change

The tactic of deploying the silent majority as shock troops to quell calls for civil rights reform has been sustained by the political right in the United States for over a half century. On the surface, the politics of backlash are the centerpiece of resistance to social justice movements in the contemporary period. However, the strategy of bombarding policy discourse with hyperbole and ad hominem attacks serves a greater purpose. It distracts attention away from the broader neoliberal agenda of the political right which is delineated by scholars like Hackworth (2019). In order to engage this agenda, we must look past the strawman that frames civil rights policies as flawed, wasteful, sectarian, left-wing folly.

Hackworth (2019) argues that efforts to dismantle civil rights legislation are at the forefront of a broader right-wing agenda to promote neoliberal policies aimed at creating a minimalist social welfare state, deregulating industry and the economy, promoting free trade, and lowering taxes. He notes that, "the key policy applications of neoliberalism – austerity, free trade, low taxes for the rich – are unpopular and most politicians do their best to cloak their implementation in some other discourse or rationale" (Hackworth, 2019, p. 54). In order to clear a path for neoliberal policies, the right-wing movement mobilized around white racial resentment. By redirecting public discourse, the movement has created an army of foot soldiers willing to fight against what is arguably their own best interests. Brown (2018, p. 74) elaborates on the dilemma created by the contemporary right-wing political movement and its implications for civil rights policies and social justice reform:

> Neoliberalism indicts the social as a fiction through which equality is pursued at the expense of the spontaneous order generated by markets and morals. It indicts the political as pretending to knowledge and making use of coercion where, in fact, ignorance prevails, and freedom should reign. A depoliticized and anti-regulatory state that also provides support for enhanced claims of the personal sphere is forwarded as the antidote to these dangers. However, the effect of this antidote is to de-democratize political culture and to discredit norms and practices of inclusion, pluralism, tolerance,

and equality across the board. Advocacy of these norms and practices is cast by neoliberal reason as a wrongheaded effort that spurns freedom, replaces morals with political mandates, and enlists the social engineering that builds totalitarianism. Hence the labeling of "social justice warriors" as "fascists" by the alt-right.

Recognizing the unpopularity of neoliberal policies, their proponents consciously pursue a path of popular disenfranchisement designed to dismantle democratic governance. It also has led to the rise of tenuous coalitions of governing partners with widely disparate views whose work together has been largely ineffective (see extended discussion in Levitsky & Ziblatt, 2019). To date, the strategy has worked. In order to reverse course, the veneer produced by backlash politics must be stripped away.

How social workers and community practitioners can respond to backlash politics

There is an urgent need for social workers, community practitioners, activists, and advocates to redouble their efforts to deconstruct backlash politics. The deployment of strategies based on backlash politics has allowed the broader neoliberal agenda to fly under the radar with limited scrutiny and accountability. This has resulted in the weakening of civil rights policies and the reproduction of inequality and discrimination in an array of social institutions – including those served by social workers (National Association of Social Workers [NASW], 2020). In this section we outline a three-pronged strategy that practitioners can use to respond to backlash politics. It entails: (1) removing the will of members of the silent majority to engage in backlash politics; (2) recruiting institutional allies to social justice movements; and (3) expanding the capacity of social justice movements in order to foster policy change and incubate new programs at the local, state, and federal levels. All three components of this strategy need to be pursued simultaneously.

Winning the hearts and minds of the silent majority

One of the ironies of the right-wing movement's southern strategy is that its goal of dismantling civil rights policies works to the detriment of disaffected whites. For instance, the Bureau of Labor Statistics has documented that contrary to widely held beliefs among the general citizenry, whites disproportionately benefit from social welfare, housing, transportation, healthcare, social security, and other public programs designed to reduce poverty (Foster & Rojas, 2018). Advocates for social justice need to redouble their efforts to highlight how the silent majority benefits from the policies it opposes. One way to achieve this is by disseminating data on social welfare program participation. Another is to support and publicize initiatives that appeal to a wide range of voters, including the silent majority. For example, most Americans support limits on the profits of pharmaceutical companies, through negotiating for the cost of prescription drugs (Hamel et al., 2021). Making the silent majority more aware of how social welfare programs benefit disaffected whites can create a wedge that allows for discourse about the detrimental effects the broader neoliberal agenda of the right has for working- and middle-class families.

It is imperative to defuse the silent majority's willingness to fight against civil rights policies. This group constitutes the shock troops of the right-wing movement. Even if the silent majority doesn't join social justice movements, convincing them to disengage from politics and remain at home to preserve self-interests that, in turn, will change the dynamic of public discourse. Without the firewall of the silent majority, proponents of neoliberal policies will be forced to make a case for their ideas out in the open. In such a forum, advocacy for austerity measures, unfettered free trade, tax cuts for the rich, political disenfranchisement, and other neoliberal policies will wither.

Collaborate with guerillas in the bureaucracy

Advocates for social justice must prioritize the development of relationships with allies in local, state, and federal governmental agencies. Moreover, with more than four out of ten employed in government, social workers have a responsibility not only to work for social justice within these agencies but also to serve as social change agents within their employing organizations (NASW Center for Workplace Studies and Social Work Practice, 2011), These individuals can disseminate information about institutional practices, provide technical support to grassroots and nonprofit organizations, and identify paths to connect the broad goals of social justice organizations with concrete poli- cies. This type of bridge building is essential to addressing the disconnect between the ideological imperative of social justice movements and the need to deliver tangible benefits to affected communities. This disconnect is identified by Szetela (2020) as a major obstacle to sustained social movements and institutional change.

When forging these relationships, leaders of social justice movements need to be diligent in identifying allies in government who are both amenable to their goals and willing to disclose information to grassroots organizers. Needleman and Needleman (1974, p. 326–327) discuss the critical role that *administrative guerrillas* can fill in community development and social justice movements. These insiders can provide community members with nonpublic information and technical assistance that, in turn, can be used to build their capacity, protect their interests, and forward their policy agendas.

In order to further this type of strategic collaboration, institutions that train professionals in fields like social work and community practice need to incorporate political agency and administrative guerrilla tactics as core component of the professional curriculum. These practices need to be embedded in codes of ethical and professional conduct for practitioners in order to transform the helping professions and disentangle them from existing institutional structures where an ethos of racism, clientelism and institutional dependence supplants community empowerment (NASW 2011). Otherwise, the concerns expressed by Piven and Cloward (1971) and Lipsky (1984) about the role of social welfare institutions in regulating and disenfranchising members of American society will endure. As noted by Reisch (2013), as long as those in social work and other helping professions continue to embrace approaches (including the training of new generations of professionals) that support the status quo by emphasizing individual adaptation, personal change and compliance while de-emphasizing resistance, social action, and social solidarity against oppressive institutional structures, we diminish opportunities to engage in meaningful structural change and dismantle racism.

Putting the policy rubber to the road

Finally, there is a need for social justice movements to increase their focus on producing tangible benefits for communities. One of the longstanding critiques of these movements is that they become prisoners of platitudes at the expense of being incubators for policy innovations. Advocates must amplify concrete policies that will lead to meaningful social change. These activities go beyond simply advocating for new laws to be passed and programs to be implemented. In addition to these activities, there is a need for movements to incubate and initiate pilot programs of their own. Consistent with Iverson's (2013) description of Do-It-Yourself activities aimed at social change, resident-driven actions, such as Reclaim Northside (Teixeira & Sing, 2016), which utilized data-driven community organizing techniques to document neighborhood blight and property abandonment in a predominantly Black neighborhood in Pittsburgh, may serve as tools for equity and racial justice in Black and Brown communities. The authors in this special issue describe pilot programs that focus on crime prevention collaborations in Langley Park, Maryland (Lung-Aman, Alvarez & Green) and fostering positive contact and relationships with returning citizens in Buffalo, New York (St. Vil & Boatley). Thurber, Bates, and Halvorson (this issue) discuss the use of community preference policies to advance racial justice and wellbeing in gentrifying neighborhoods in Portland, Oregon. Finally, preliminary findings from two different types of leadership programs aimed at training Black and Brown leaders at the intersection of politics, race and policy are discussed (Douglas-Glenn, Marlowe, Shaheen & Faulks; Chupp, Crawford Fletcher & Graulty).

In the existing neoliberal institutional milieu, civil rights and social welfare programs are systematically blocked and stunted at the federal and state levels (Lipsky, 1984). There is a pressing need for existing policies to be augmented at the local level. Advocacy groups need to incubate and design programs that can be piloted at the local level in order to generate models that can be replicated and scaled-up elsewhere. In this way, social justice movements can drive policy innovation by delivering concrete benefits to communities on the ground. Although they might find inspiration from existing policies and programs across the United States and in other countries, local social justice movements need to take the lead in policy innovation and pilot novel programs. Recent examples from Detroit, Michigan include the resident opposition to Project Green Light, the Detroit Police Department's surveillance program which led to the 2019 rescission of the use of facial recognition technology and enhanced accountability for the misuse of data and technology. Moreover, a coalition of residents, community activists and community groups championed the creation of the Detroiters' Bill of Rights which addresses issues such as "affordable water and housing, disability rights, safety, immigration rights, and a right to recreation and quality of life" (Petty, 2021, p. 7) as part of the revised City Charter. The revised charter proposes the establishment of Offices for Immigrant Affairs and Disability Affairs, restructuring of the Board of Police Commissioners, and the demilitarization of the police. These examples highlight how the incubation of social justice reforms at the local level can form a reservoir of policy options to be drawn from for broader adoption.

ORCID

Robert Mark Silverman ⓘD http://orcid.org/0000-0003-2155-7871

References

Bennett, L. (1993). Harold Washington and the black urban regime. *Urban Affairs Quarterly*, *28*(3), 423–440. https://doi.org/10.1177/004208169302800304

Boussac, T. (2021). Conservative populism and the American welfare state since the 1960s. In K. Tournier-Sol & M. Gayte (Eds.), *The faces of contemporary populism in Western Europe and the US* (pp. 181–201). Palgrave Macmillan.

Boychuk, G. W. (2008). *National health insurance in the United States and Canada: Race, territory, and the roots of difference*. Georgetown University Press.

Brown, H. E. (2013). Race, legality, and the social policy consequences of anti-immigration mobilization. *American Sociological Review*, *78*(2), 290–314. https://doi.org/10.1177/0003122413476712

Brown, W. (2018). Neoliberalism's Frankenstein: Authoritarian freedom in twenty-first century "democracies. *Critical Times*, *1*(1), 60–79. https://doi.org/10.1215/26410478-1.1.60

Enos, R. D., Kaufman, A. R., & Sands, M. L. (2019). Can violent protest change local policy support?: Evidence from the aftermath of the 1992 Los Angeles riot. *American Political Science Review*, *113*(4), 1012–1028. https://doi.org/10.1017/S0003055419000340

Feagin, J. R., & Hohle, R. (2017). *Racism in the neoliberal era: A meta history of elite white power*. Routledge.

Foster, A. C., & Rojas, A. (2018, January). Program participation and spending patterns of families receiving government means-tested assistance, *Monthly Labor Review*, 50–71. U.S. Bureau of Labor Statistics. https://www.bls.gov/opub/mlr/2018/article/program-participation-and-spending-patterns-of-families-receiving-means-tested-assistance.htm

Friesema, H. P. (1969). Black control of central cities: The hollow prize. *Journal of the American Institute of Planners, 35*(2), 75–79. https://doi.org/10.1080/01944366908977576

Glickman, N. (2020, May 21). How white backlash controls American progress: Backlash dynamics are one of the defining patterns of the county's history. *The Atlantic*, 1–13. https://www.theatlantic.com/ideas/archive/2020/05/white-backlash-nothing-new/611914/

Gordon-Reed, A. (2021). *On Juneteenth*. W. W. Norton.

Hackworth, J. (2019). Urban crisis as conservative bonding capital. *City, 23*(1), 63–75. https://doi.org/10.1080/13604813.2019.1575116

Hamel, L., Lopes, L., Kirzinger, A., Sparks, G., Kearney, A., Stokes, M., & Brodie, M. (2021 June 15). Public opinion on prescription drugs and their prices. https://www.kff.org/health-costs/poll-finding/public-opinion-on-prescription-drugs-and-their-prices/

Iverson, K. (2013). Cities within the city: Do-It-Yourself urbanism and the right to the city. *International Journal of Urban and Regional Research, 37*(3), 941–956. https://doi.org/10.1111/1468-2427.12053

Johnson, C. (2016). The half-life of the Black urban regime. *Labor Studies Journal, 41*(3), 248–255. https://doi.org/10.1177/0160449X16652981

Katz, M. B. (1990). *The undeserving poor: From the war on poverty to the war on welfare*. Pantheon.

Kraus, N., & Swanstrom, T. (2001). Minority mayors and the hollow-prize problem. *Political Science and Politics, 34*(1), 99–105. https://doi.org/10.1017/S1049096501000154

Lane, K., Williams, Y., Hunt, A. N., & Paulk, A. (2020). The framing of race: Trayvon martin and the black lives matter movement. *Journal of Black Studies, 51*(8), 790–812. https://doi.org/10.1177/0021934720946802

Levine, M. (2018, July 23). The deserving and undeserving poor: A persistent frame with consequences. *Nonprofit Quarterly*. https://nonprofitquarterly.org/the-deserving-and-undeserving-poor-a-persistent-frame-with-consequences/

Levitsky, S., & Ziblatt, D. (2019). *How democracies die*. Penguin Books.

Lipsky, M. (1984). Bureaucratic disentitlement in social welfare programs. *Social Service Review, 58*(1), 3–27. https://doi.org/10.1086/644161

Maxwell, A., & Shields, T. (2014). The fate of Obamacare: Racial resentment, ethnocentrism and attitudes about healthcare reform. *Race and Social Problems, 6*(4), 293–304. https://doi.org/10.1007/s12552-014-9130-5

Milner, A., & Franz, B. (2020). Anti-black attitudes are a threat to health equity in the United States. *Journal of Racial and Ethnic Health Disparities, 7*(1), 169–176. https://doi.org/10.1007/s40615-019-00646-0

Murray, C. (1985). *Losing ground: American social policy 1950-1980*. Basic Books.

NASW (2011). Social workers in government agencies: Occupational profiles. https://www.socialworkers.org/LinkClick.aspx?fileticket=Uxvwi_qOumU%3D&portalid=0

National Association of Social Workers. (2020, August 21). *Social workers must help dismantle systems of oppression and fight racism within social work profession*. https://www.socialworkers.org/News/News-Releases/ID/2219/Social-Workers-Must-Help-Dismantle-Systems-of-Oppression-and-Fight-Racism-Within-Social-Work-Profession

Needleman, M. L., & Needleman, C. E. (1974). *Guerrillas in the bureaucracy: The community planning experiment in the United States*. John Wiley & Sons.

Owens, M. L. (2020). The urban world is a world of police. *Journal of Race, Ethnicity and the City, 1*(1–2), 11–15. https://doi.org/10.1080/26884674.2020.1795488

Peterson, P. E., & Rom, M. C. (1990). *Welfare magnets: A new case for a national standard.* Brookings Institution Press.

Petty, T. (2021 March 5). Detroit on a journey to be seen. *Data for Black Lives.* https://blog.d4bl.org/detroit-on-a-journey-to-be-seen-2/

Piven, F. F., & Cloward, R. A. (1971). *Regulating the poor: The functions of public welfare.* Pantheon Books.

Reed, A. (1988). The black urban regime: Structural origins and constraints. (M. P. Smith, Ed.). *community and the city* (pp. 138–189). Transaction Books.

Reisch, M. (2013). Social work education and the neo-liberal challenge: The US response to increasing global inequality. *Social Work Education, 32*(6), 715–733. https://doi.org/10.1080/02615479.2013.809200

Rieder, J. (1989). The rise of the "silent majority." In S. Fraeser& & G. Gerstle (Eds.), *The rise and fall of the New Deal order, 1930-1980* (pp. 243–268). Princeton University Press.

Santiago, A. M. (2015). Fifty years later: From a war on poverty to a war on the poor. *Social Problems, 62*(1), 2–14. https://doi.org/10.1093/socpro/spu009

Santiago, A. M., & Ivery, J. (2020). Removing the knees from their necks: Mobilizing community practice and social action for racial justice. *Journal of Community Practice, 28*(3), 195–207. https://doi.org/10.1080/10705422.2020.1823672

Sekou, B. D. (2020). The limits of black politics in the post-civil rights era. *Sociological Forum, 35*(S1), 954–973. https://doi.org/10.1111/socf.12602

Silverman, R. M., & Patterson, K. L. (2012). The four horsemen of the fair housing apocalypse: A critique of fair housing policy in the USA. *Critical Sociology, 38*(1), 123–140. https://doi.org/10.1177/0896920510396385

Silverman, R. M., Patterson, K. L., & Wang, C. (2021). Questioning stereotypes about US site-based subsidized housing. *International Journal of Housing Markets and Analysis, 14*(3), 613–631. https://doi.org/10.1108/IJHMA-05-2020-0057

Szetela, A. (2020). Black Lives Matter at five: Limits and possibilities. *Ethnic and Racial Studies, 43*(8), 1358–1383. https://doi.org/10.1080/01419870.2019.1638955

Teixeira, S., & Sing, E. (2016). Reclaim Northside: An environmental justice approach to address vacant land in Pittsburgh. *Family and Community Health, 39*(3), 207–215. http://dx.doi.org/10.1097/FCH.0000000000000107

Wasow, O. (2020). Agenda seeding: How 1960s black protests moved elites, public opinion and voting. *American Political Science Review, 114*(3), 638–659. https://doi.org/10.1017/S000305542000009X

Wilson, W. J. (1990). *The truly disadvantaged: The inner city, the underclass, and public policy.* University of Chicago Press.

Zolberg, A. (1999). Matters of state: Theorizing immigration policy (C. Hirschman, P. Kasinitz, & J. DeWind, Eds.). *The handbook of international migration: The American experience* (pp. 71–93). Russell Sage Foundation.

Removing the knees from their necks: mobilizing community practice and social action for racial justice

Anna Maria Santiago and Jan Ivery

In the midst of a year of seemingly insurmountable struggles associated with the COVID-19 pandemic, the United States and other countries across the globe are grappling with another deadly pandemic responsible for taking untold lives and destroying the health, well-being and potential of millions of people and the communities in which they reside. This pandemic – systemic racism – is not new. For 400 years, systemic racism (also known as institutionalized or structural racism) has been used in the United States primarily against African Americans as an institutionalized mechanism of social control, economic exploitation, and white supremacy. Systemic racism manifests itself in a myriad of interconnected ways, including disparities in health, education, employment, and housing; voter suppression; and disproportionate exposure to state-sanctioned violence at the hands of law enforcement (Bonilla-Silva, 2018; Dettlaff, 2020; Edwards, Lee & Esposito, 2019; Lavalette & Penketh, 2014; National Association of Social Workers (NASW), 2020a; Schwartz, 2020). Further, systemic racism and the disregard for civil rights and equal protection it produces has underscored how little Black lives continue to matter to those in power (Abrams & Detlaff, 2020; Cobbina, 2019; Newman, 2015). Over time, the devaluation and dehumanization of certain segments of U.S. society extended to other minoritized groups, such as Latinx and Indigenous Peoples, who share similar experiences of over-criminalization, over-punishment, and exposure to discriminatory practices (Bonilla-Silva, 2018; Corral, 2020; Council on Social Work Education (CSWE), 2020; Jean, 2020; Rios et al., 2020; Schroedel & Chin, 2020). *Systemic racism is both an invisible and visible knee on the necks of Black, Brown, and Indigenous people in this country.*

Bonilla-Silva (2018) and others (for Fekete, 2014; Lavalette & Penketh, 2014; Newman, 2015; Singh, 2011, 2014) contend that not only has systemic racism permeated the values, attitudes and structures of society, it has worsened over the past 40 years. At the same time, however, racist actions and behaviors not only have become more pervasive, they also have become less overt, more subtle and hidden. According to Bonilla-Silva (2018), colorblind racism surfaced in the post-Civil

Rights era with proponents attempting to explain away existing racial inequalities as artifacts of market dynamics and cultural limitations. Almost as troubling as the enduring presence of systemic racism, however, is the growth of social and political movements in the United States and beyond that seek to discredit its existence altogether (Trainin Blank, n.d.). New political contexts, evident in the nativist and Far Alt-Right movements emerging in the United States, countries throughout Europe, and Australia, add to the complexity of current dynamics on race wherein racial inequities are increasingly denied or couched using color-neutral terms. *Denying the existence of racial inequalities is a knee on the necks of Black, Brown, and Indigenous people in this country.*

Systemic racism in the U.S. context

Numerous observations have been made about systemic racism in the U.S. context (see for example, Allen-Meares & Burman, 1995; Bonilla-Silva, 2018; Carten, 2016; Cobbina, 2019; Cramer & Smith McElveen, 2003; Jean, 2020; Newman, 2015). Twenty-five years ago, Allen-Meares and Burman (1995) suggested that Americans resided in a "nation strained by racism, hostility and hatred" (p. 268). However, Cramer and Smith McElveen (2003) also noted that in the shift toward "multiculturalism, pluralism and diversity . . . matters of race were diluted or lost" (p. 43). Bonilla-Silva (2018) maintained that the transition to more subtle, implicit racism is linked to ideology casting U.S. social institutions as neutral, post-racial and colorblind. Likewise, embedded within U.S. political systems are elected officials and community leaders who have a penchant for gaslighting or discrediting the concerns of U.S. citizens about systemic racism and state-sanctioned violence toward African Americans and other minoritized communities.

Yet, these attempts at gaslighting fall flat in the face of evidence increasingly captured by social media (Cobbina, 2019). We have seen African Americans from all social class backgrounds and across different localities harassed or threatened while engaging in activities of daily living. Every day, numerous videos are posted on social media depicting acts of vigilantism perpetrated by neighbors or violence committed by law enforcement against African Americans. Rios et al. (2020) report similar patterns of harassment and threats by the police in working-class Latinx neighborhoods. During the past few years, overt acts of police violence against minoritized communities in the United States, the United Kingdom, and Australia have garnered global attention and notoriety (Fox et al., 2019; Krakouer, 2020; Long, 2018) as these images of brutality are transmitted worldwide via social media. Contemporary examples of vigilante beatings, police shootings, or chokeholds have become the modern-day equivalents to the lynchings that Ida B. Wells Barnett (1901) argued were used to strip African Americans of their civil rights and humanity while asserting power and terror (McDermott, 2018; Squire,

2020). *Vigilantism and police brutality are the knees on the necks of Black, Brown and Indigenous people in this country.*

A lingering concern is the growing disconnect between the vivid images capturing the use of deadly force by the police and official reports of such events. Indeed, a major critique of law enforcement has been the lack of transparency and record-keeping (Newman, 2015). The U.S. Federal Bureau of Investigation and other federal law enforcement bodies lack nationwide tracking systems to document police-involved shootings. To compensate, there are several public databases, such as the Fatal Encounters database and Mapping Police Violence, that have been compiled by researchers or journalists to document these shootings. According to Mapping Police Violence, a total of 7,641 fatal police shootings were documented during the period between 2013 and 2019 (Mapping Police Violence, n.d.). Of the 12,300 police departments in the country (Bureau of Justice Statistics, 2019), more than 2,500 police departments – one out of five – employed officers who shot and killed at least one person during the past five years (Fox et al., 2019).

Nearly 26% of the victims of fatal police shootings were African American, 18% were Latinx, and 3% were Indigenous (Mapping Police Violence, n.d.). The percentage of fatal police shootings of Latinos was slightly higher than the percentage of Latinos in the overall population; however, these percentages were approximately twice at high for African Americans and Indigenous people. Likewise, police shootings were identified as a leading cause of death for African American men. In a recent study of violent encounters with police, Edwards, Lee and Esposito, (2019) found that African American men were 2.5 times more likely to be shot and killed by police than White men. Surprisingly, African American women were 1.4 times more likely to killed by police than White men. Compared to White men, Indigenous men were 1.2–1.7 times and Latinx men were 1.4 times more likely to be killed by police (Edwards et al., 2019). These heightened risks of being killed by police remained over the life course. Moreover, unarmed African Americans were more likely to be killed by police using aggressive approaches or excessive use of force; indeed, one-third of unarmed victims of police shootings involved Black citizens (Fox et al., 2019; Schwartz, 2020). As Newman (2015, p. 124) notes, the police and the institutions that support them, have normalized the killing of Black unarmed men. Although the number of fatal police shootings has been trending downward for Whites since 2013, it continues trending upward for people of color (Mapping Police Violence, n.d.). *The sheer number of police shootings and the lack of accountability for them are knees on the necks of Black, Brown and Indigenous people in this country.*

Witnessing shootings of African American men and women by the police firsthand or by social media, provide frequent and concrete illustrations of deeply embedded patterns of racial hostility within police departments (Cobbina, 2019). At the same time citizens, particularly those of color, view the legal system in the United States with great skepticism since it allows police to operate with impunity and limited accountability (Newman, 2015). It is no wonder that minority men and women express frequent concerns for themselves and their children about the potential of being victims of police violence. Many minority parents engage in "the talk" about interactions with police with their adolescent children in the hopes of minimizing the risk of any life-threatening encounters. Unlike White adults, African American and Latinx adults from all social class backgrounds are vigilant in terms of protecting themselves and their families from police brutality. In a recent national study of African American, Latinx and White adults, Graham et al. (2020) found that 70% of African American and 64% of Latino respondents were concerned about experiencing police brutality. In contrast, 75% of Whites respondents indicated that they were not worried about police brutality at all. When controlling for factors that might affect these concerns, African Americans were 5.3 times more likely to worry about police brutality and Latinos 4 times more likely as compared to White study participants (Graham et al., 2020).

Unfortunately, their worries are not unfounded. Racialized notions of criminal propensity and suspicion – guilty until proven innocent – are attached to members of minority groups by the larger society. Additionally, these are further applied to criminalize poor communities of color (Rios et al., 2020). These stereotypes provide common justifications for the deaths of African Americans, Latinx and Indigenous people in police custody (Cobbina, 2019; Long, 2018). As Long (2018) notes, widespread racial tropes cast Black people, and, we argue by extension, other minorities as perpetual suspects even when they are victims of crime. Common public recriminations reverberate in commentaries such as "S/he would not have been shot if they were not doing anything wrong" or "S/he should have followed what the police officers were telling them to do." Yet, videos of events ranging from harassment during everyday activities to those capturing George Floyd's arrest and death underscore the deleterious effects that these racialized responses have on the health and well-being of individuals, their families, and their communities. *The inability to live everyday lives without fear of police brutality is a knee on the neck of Black, Brown and Indigenous people in this country.*

These and other well-publicized acts of police violence have elicited widespread condemnation from governments, organizations and individuals worldwide, including social work professionals (Abrams & Detlaff, 2020; Cherry, 2020; Dettlaff, 2020) and professional organizations (CSWE, 2020; Grand Challenges for Social Work, 2020; NASW, 2007, 2020a, 2020b). Moreover, they have resulted in worldwide protests against the injustice experienced by Black men and women and the growing rejection of how police criminalize groups of people in society (Cobbina, 2019; Evans et al., 2020; Moore et al., 2016). Protesters may feel a sense of duty or responsibility to get involved in the fight against racism and wish to become part of the movement to address inequities in not only the criminal justice system but also in education, employment and housing (see Cobbina, 2019). Newman (2015, p. 127) argues that protests occur when "citizens believe the criminal justice system has failed and police officers were not held accountable for their actions". *Communities and their citizens are clamoring for our social institutions to remove the knee of racial injustice from the necks of Black, Brown and Indigenous people in this country.*

Social work as a knee on the necks of Black, Brown and Indigenous peoples

At different points in the history of social work and social welfare in the United States, including the unprecedented times in which we are living, collective soul-searching within the profession has raised the question: *Is social work and, by extension, the social work profession racist*? Not surprisingly, the results of that soul-searching have produced a resounding yes (Abrams & Detlaff, 2020; Allen-Meares & Burman, 1995; McMahon & Allen-Meares, 1992; NASW, 2007; Trolander, 1997). In the early 1990s, McMahon and Allen-Meares offered a searing rebuke to the profession – identifying social workers as controlling, coercive, and racist while employed in organizations and systems that provided differential treatment to clients. Others have reminded us of the ways in which social work and social welfare have been complicit in maintaining systemic racism and the status quo (Allen-Meares & Burman, 1995; Carten, 2016; Cherry, 2020; Miller et al., 2004; Ring, 2012). Over the years, the social work profession has been coopted into racist and discriminatory practices and processes through a duty of surveillance (Lavalette & Penketh, 2014; Miller et al., 2004).

Allen-Meares and Burman (1995) referred to social workers as agents of social control who remained silent about the "inequities and social conditions affecting African American families" (see pp. 270–271). This denigration of and disrespect toward minority families by the profession was echoed further by Abrams and Detlaff (2020):

> "As a profession, we have not yet reckoned with the racism and anti-Blackness that exists among ourselves and our key social welfare institutions, including public benefits and child welfare ... Need to recognize social work's historical role in perpetuating anti-Blackness" (para #1).

Recently, the National Association of Social Workers (NASW) acknowledged the longstanding influence of racism and white supremacy on social work practice and ideology (NASW, 2020b). In particular, NASW singles out the child welfare system that "more rigorously regulated and castigated Black, Brown, and Indigenous families" (para. #3) as well as the role that social workers played in perpetuating these harmful systems. Continued differential treatment of minority families, particularly African American families, prompted Holosko et al. (2017) to ask: *Do Black lives matter to social work?*

Policy documents disclose considerable vacillation over the years by social work professional associations regarding their responsibilities toward addressing racism in their organizations and activities as well as within accredited social work training programs. Although CSWE adopted its first policy banning racial discrimination within the organization in 1961, support for antidiscrimination waned by the mid-1970s as the organization became more conservative and racist (see discussion in Trolander, 1997). Responding to racism and white supremacy in the profession, the National Association of Black Social Workers (NABSW) disengaged from the National Conference on Social Welfare in 1968 in order to address issues of racism and poverty in America and advocate for systemic change (National Association of Black Social Workers, n.d.). In 2005, the NASW adopted its policy statement on racism which enjoined all social workers "to recognize and confront all forms of racism" (NASW, 2020a, p. 3). This was subsequently echoed in the NASW report, *Institutional racism & the social work profession: A call to action* (NASW, 2007) which challenged the "profession to have the courage to label racism as racism" (p. 23) and provided an extensive roadmap to address systemic racism within the profession and the larger society. Despite these directives, social workers tended to view racism as something located outside of the profession while continuing to ignore the extent to which aversive racism permeated social work training programs and organizations (Ring, 2012). Moreover, the country's longstanding history of racism and discriminatory legislation reproduced a two-track, separate but unequal social service delivery system that social workers were instrumental in operating (Carten, 2016).

Additional concerns have been raised about the role that systemic racism plays in social work education and research. In addition to the documents developed by the national social work professional organizations, other scholars point to the lack of alignment between clinical social work training, practice, and the profession's mission of racial justice in service to marginalized and oppressed groups (Sakamoto, 2007; Smith, 2019; Varghese, 2018). Despite the heavy emphasis on cultural competence and diversity training, faculty and practitioners suggest that "social work students are not challenged enough to think critically about race and ethnocentrism" (see for example, Krakouer, 2020, para #9). Further, Edmonds-Cady and Wingfield (2017) contend that social work educators reinforce systemic racism.

On the research side, McMahon and Allen-Meares (1992) were among the first social work educators to assess social work scholarship on race. In their review of top social work journals, they found few manuscripts that addressed racism experienced by minoritized groups. Also, missing from the published literature was research on institutional change to reduce structural inequalities. They note a general reluctance to promote social action using community or macro practice. Replicating the methods used by McMahon and Allen-Meares in their earlier study, Corley and Young (2018) found a lack of attention, involvement, and inaction on issues of racial injustice. They contend that "if social workers are failing to address systemic racial inequities, they are complicit in their maintenance" (p. 318). Both studies argue that social work discussions of racial oppression seem to pay lip service to structural issues that perpetuate systemic racism. They also suggest that social work research replicates the "apartheid of knowledge in academia" (p. 323). Yet, social work researchers can and have exacerbated distrust when they have approached minority communities as their own personal laboratories extracting knowledge with little or no reciprocity or regard for those affected (Edmonds-Cady & Wingfield, 2017). Finally, despite the call to identifying racism as one of the profession's grand challenges (see Davis, 2016), it wasn't until June 2020 that the Grand Challenges for Social Work (2020) added eradicating racism as the thirteenth area of concern for social work scholars and educators.

Removing the knees from their necks: Adopting anti-racist social work

Anti-racist social work appeared in the United Kingdom, Canada and Australia in the 1970s and 1980s (Lavalette & Penketh, 2014). In the United Kingdom, concerns about systemic racism led to the development of anti-racist social work practice in the 1980s and 1990s (Lavalette & Penketh, 2014). Instead of focusing exclusively on addressing individual prejudices, the purpose of anti-racist social work was to expose the structural and institutional nature of racism embedded in British society and challenge oppressive practices and structures in the workplace and in communities (Penketh & Lavalette, 2014). Anti-racist social workers recognized that racism also permeated social services, service delivery systems and social work education. Members of the movement focused on promoting municipal level social change and introducing anti-discrimination policies and practices within social work education and social care organizations. These activities produced promising effects on municipal level social change as well as changes in the profession (Lavalette & Penketh, 2014; Singh, 2014).

More recently, Fekete (2014), writing about Britain, describes another form of systemic racism that arose since the late 1990s – that of *xeno-racism* or fear of the other – supporting institutionalized actions and behaviors that devalue or target particular groups on the basis of attributes that are used to define their "otherness," such as class, political affiliation, nationality, culture or religion. Xeno-racism can be applied to groups that are identified as racially White. For example, this leads to everyday aggression in public spaces toward people speaking a language other than English as well as terrorist activities such as the bombing of mosques. While it is clear that xeno-racism constitutes a form of oppression in the United States, eliminating systemic racism against Black, Brown and Indigenous bodies needs to be a priority for social work.

By the beginning of the 21st century, the anti-racism movement within social work in Britain was replaced by an emphasis on diversity, equality and cultural competence – a move that Jeyasingham and Morton (2019) argues was utilized to provide superficial evidence of social equality. One of the unfinished tasks of the anti-racist social work movement in Britain was changing the culture and structure of organizations (Singh, 2011). Fekete (2014) suggests that despite movement toward greater equity, the social work profession remained uncomfortable with anti-racism strategies that sought to move more deeply into structural change of British social institutions.

Unlike the United Kingdom, a comparable anti-racist social work movement did not take root in the United States (see Reisch & Andrews, 2002). Instead, social work professional organizations in the United States avoided a critical analysis of institutional and structural discrimination and oppression to concentrate on individual development of cultural competence by social workers in order to facilitate their work with minority clients and communities. Lavalette and Penketh (2014) suggest that the profession's focus on cultural competence and its most recent iteration, diversity, was less risky politically. Perhaps an unintended consequence, the use of "cultural competence otherizes non-whites without having to invoke racist language" (Pon, 2009, p. 62). More recently, social work has examined the potential of the anti-oppression approach to practice with individuals and communities (see for example, Morgaine & Capous-Desyllas, 2014). However, this approach, which has been applied to a wide array of underrepresented groups, may dilute efforts to address systemic racism precisely because it de-emphasizes the specific contexts underlying racial inequalities experienced by African Americans and others in the United States.

Mobilizing community practice and social action for racial justice

The social work profession must address systemic racism as part of our mandate to "promote change from within and among organizations and society" (NASW, 2007, p. 3). A first step is to recognize systemic racism and its various manifestations within the profession. Until social work is able critically analyze how the profession and social work curricula perpetuate racism, the profession will be limited in its ability to implement the change needed to eradicate it in our institutions. As Cherry (2020, p. 1) notes, the "failure to take explicit action to promote race equity is equivalent to maintaining and supporting oppressive and racist systems." Identifying and acknowledging systemic racism is a critical first step but it is not enough. We need to take deliberate actions to confront all forms of racism, both overt and subtle, within all of the institutions that undergird our profession (NASW,

2007, p. 3). To do so, social work must disrupt established practices that continue to support and promote white privilege. This includes the need for all to examine how their attitudes and behaviors uphold racism.

Social workers can and must take actions to reverse the effect of racism on service delivery in Black, Brown and Indigenous communities. Social workers must challenge their organizations to become antiracist organizations and upend the status quo. Part of challenging the status quo involves developing systems and structures that are inclusive and equitable. However, inclusion alone is insufficient for addressing the deep-seated social ills associated with racism (Miller, 2020). In real world implementation, inclusion requires the membership cost of conformity. To achieve this, organizations and institutions must create mechanisms whereby diversity is inherently embodied, pragmatically instituted and consistently ensured. By doing so, diversity normalizes difference instead of "othering" it.

Moving forward the profession needs to get its own house in order before trying to insert itself into current discussions about dismantling systemic racism in the nation's criminal justice system. As Abrams and Detlaff (2020) stated so eloquently, " Social work cannot situate itself as the magic ingredient to eradicating racism in law enforcement if we cannot dismantle racism within our own systems of care" (para #2). Among potential remedies to address police brutality in minority communities that are currently under consideration is the addition of social workers to police crisis intervention teams – something that has been implemented on a small scale already. Also, mandatory training of police on the use of de-escalation techniques and trauma-informed responses during crises warrants further deliberation and action; this training can be performed by social workers or other mental health professionals (Evans et al., 2020). The development of diversion programs whereby individuals needing access to mental health services are referred to those services instead of incarceration deserves further consideration. Recent proposals suggesting the replacement of police by social workers seem less plausible than the scaffolding of mental health and social services and other alternatives to incarceration within communities to support individuals during crises thereby diminishing the need for law enforcement intervention.

Since the death of George Floyd at the hands of police in Minneapolis (MN), the Black Lives Matter movement has recommended the dismantling and disinvestment of the police – actions that have been endorsed by a small, but growing number of municipalities in the United States. Petitions to remove school resource officers from public schools are also gaining traction. Rampant police brutality clearly underscores that our criminal justice system is not serving the people whose hard-earned taxes keep it afloat. We support calls to end government-sanctioned excessive use of force and mass incarceration. We also urge lawmakers in the Senate to deliberate the George Floyd Justice in Policing Act of 2020 (HR 7120) and pursue meaningful police reform.

We also support efforts to develop community-driven alternatives for public safety – community members need to be shaping the policing occurring in their neighborhoods and prioritizing local safety needs. The composition of local police commissions and human relations commissions need to reflect the communities they serve and function independently from police unions or municipal leaders. Community practitioners can play important roles in working with community residents to amplify their voices. Activities promoting voter registration and getting out the vote as well as vigorously protecting voting rights are critical to removing the knee from the necks of Black, Brown, and Indigenous people.

Further, we support calls to reinvest in our communities in order to create opportunity structures and pathways for all, and especially our most vulnerable citizens, to realize their full potential. Practitioners can facilitate the use of asset-based community development (ABCD) approaches as they work with community members to design and implement community-led initiatives supporting residents across the life span.

Finally, we support the development and dissemination of scholarship focusing on racial justice in Black, Brown and Indigenous communities. We encourage scholars to engage in collaborative research with communities of color, conduct comparative analysis between the United States and other countries when possible, or apply critical race theory to the study of inequality. This also means supporting scholars of color who conduct this research. A special issue of the *Journal of Community Practice* is already under development. Look for *Beyond Lip Service: Bringing Racial Justice to Black and Brown Communities* in late 2021.

As we navigate these unchartered waters or social change, may we remind one another that Black lives will not truly matter until we act in tangible ways to ensure that they do.

Acknowledgement

This editorial benefited from helpful comments from JCP Co-Editor Richard J. Smith. He would like readers to know that he supports the recommendations for social work and community practice made in the editorial.

References

Abrams, L. S., & Detlaff, A. (2020, June 18). *An open letter to NASW and allied organizations on social work's relationship with law enforcement.* https://medium.com/@alandettlaff/an-open-letter-to-nasw-and-allied-organizations-on-social-works-relationship-with-law-enforcement-1a1926c71b28#:~:text=An%20Open%20Letter%20to%20NASW%20and%

20Allied%20Organizations,submitted%20these%20to%20NASW%20on%20June%2022%2C%202020

Allen-Meares, P., & Burman, S. (1995). The endangerment of African American men: An appeal for social work action [comments on currents]. *Social Work, 40*(2), 268–274.

Bonilla-Silva, E. (2018). *Racism without racists: Color blind racism and the persistence of racial inequality in America* (5th ed.). Rowman & Littlefield.

Bureau of Justice Statistics. (2019, October). *Local police departments, 2016: Personnel.* https://www.bjs.gov/content/pub/pdf/lpd16p.pdf

Carten, A. (2016, August 21). *How racism has shaped welfare policy in America since 1935. The Conversation.* https://theconversation.com/how-racism-has-shaped=welfare-policy-in - america-since-1935-63574

Cherry, L. (2020, May). Social workers: Allies for justice? *The New Social Worker Magazine.* https://www.socialworker.com/feature-articles/practice/social-workers-allies-justice/

Cobbina, J. E. (2019). *Hands up, don't shoot: Why the protests in Ferguson and Baltimore matter, and how they changed America.* New York University Press.

Corley, N. A., & Young, S. M. (2018). Is social work still racist? A content analysis of recent literature. *Social Work, 63*(4), 317–326. https://doi.org/10.1093/sw/swy042

Corral, A. J. (2020). Allies, antagonist, or ambivalent? Exploring Latino attitudes about the Black lives matter movement. *Hispanic Journal of Behavioral Sciences*, 1–24. https://doi.org/10.1177/0739986320949540

Council on Social Work Education. (2020, June 2). *CSWE statement on social justice.* https://www.cswe.org/News/Press-Room/CSWE-Statement-on-Social-Justice

Cramer, D. N., & Smith McElveen, J. (2003). Undoing racism in social work practice. *Race, Gender and Class, 10*(2), 41–57. https://www.jstor.org/stable/41675072

Davis, L. E. (2016). Race: America's grand challenge. *Journal of the Society for Social Work and Research, 7*(2), 395–403. https://doi.org/10.1086/686296

Dettlaff, A. (2020, July). *A call to act against racism and white supremacy now.* The New Social Worker. https://www.socialworker.com/feature-articles/practice/call-to-social-workers-act-against-racism-white-supremacy/

Edmonds-Cady, C., & Wingfield, T. T. (2017). Social workers: Agents of change or agents of oppression? *Social Work Education, 36*(4), 430–442. https://doi.org/10.1080/02615479.2017.1291802

Edwards, F., Lee, H., & Esposito, M. (2019). Risk of being killed by police use-of-force in the U.S. by age, race/ ethnicity,and sex. *Proceedings of the National Academy of Sciences.* https://www.pnas.org/cgi/doi/10.1073/pnas.1821204116

Evans, A. C., Jr., Levin, S., & McClain, A. (2020, August 18). Mental health leaders: We must end pandemic of racism. *Orlando Sentinel: Tribune Media.* https://www.orlandosentinel.com/opinion/guest-commentary/os-op-end-racism-pandemic-mental-health-leaders-20200818-72bfy4chubfvvbsnbiplx3yxva-story.html

Fekete, L. (2014). The growth of xeno-racism and Islamaphobia in Britain. In M. Lavalette & L. Penketh (Eds.), *Race, racism and social work: Contemporary issues and debates* (pp. 33–51). Bristol, UK: Polity Press.

Fox, J., Blanco, A., Jenkins, J., Tate, J., & Lowery, W. (2019, August 9). What we've learned about police shootings 5 years after Ferguson. *Washington Post.* https://www.washingtonpost.com/nation/2019/08/09/what-weve-learned-about-police-shootingsyears-after-ferguson/?arc404=true&itid=lk_inline_manual_19

Graham, A., Haner, M., Sloan, M. M., Cullen, F. T., Teresa, C., Kulig, T. C., & Jonson, C. L. (2020). Race and worrying about police brutality: The hidden injuries of minority status in America. *Victims & Offenders, 15*(5), 549–573. https://doi.org/10.1080/15564886.2020.1767252

Grand Challenges for Social Work. (2020, June 26). *Announcing the grand challenge to eliminate racism.* https://grandchallengesforsocialwork.org/grand-challenges-for-social-work/announcing-the-grand-challenge-to-eliminate-racism/

Holosko, M. J., Briggs, H. E., & Miller, K. M. (2017). Do black lives really matter—to social work? Introduction to the special edition. *Research on Social Work Practice, 28*(3), 272–274. https://doi.org/1049731517706551

Jean, T. (2020, June 16). *Black lives matter: Police brutality in the era of COVID-19.* Lerner Center for Health Promotion, Syracuse University. https://lernercenter.syr.edu/wp-content/uploads/2020/06/Jean.pdf

Jeyasingham, D., & Morton, J. (2019). How is 'racism' understood in literature about black and minority ethnic social work students in Britain? A conceptual review. *Social Work Education, 38*(5), 563–575. https://doi.org/10.1080/02615479.2019.1584176

Krakouer, J. (2020, August 20). Racism still exists in social work today – We need more black faces in the profession. *The Guardian.* https://www.theguardian.com/commentisfree/2020/aug/20/racism-still-exists-in-social-work-today-we-need-more-black-faces-in-the-profession

Lavalette, M., & Penketh, L. (Eds). (2014). *Race, racism and social work: Contemporary issues and debates.* Bristol, UK: Polity Press.

Long, L. (2018). *Perpetual suspects: A critical race theory of Black and mixed-raceexperiences of policing.* London: Palgrave Macmillan.

Mapping Police Violence. (n.d.). *National trends.* https://mappingpoliceviolence.org/nationaltrends

McDermott, S. P. (2018, August 22). *Jane Addams, Ida B. Wells, and racial injustice in America.* Jane Addams Papers Project. https://janeaddams.ramapo.edu/2018/08/jane-addams-ida-b-wells-and-racial-injustice-in-america

McMahon, A., & Allen-Meares, P. (1992). Is social work racist? A content analysis of recent literature. *Social Work, 37*(6), 533–539.

Miller, J. (2020, July). Beyond inclusion initiatives, toward expansive frameworks. *The New Social Worker.* https://www.socialworkers.com/feature-articles/practice/beyond-inclusion-initiatives-toward-expansive-frameworks/

Miller, J., Hyde, C. A., & Ruth, B. J. (2004). Teaching about race and racism in social work: Challenges for White educators. *Smith College Studies in Social Work, 74*(2), 409–426. https://doi.org/10.1080/00377310409517724

Moore, S. E., Robinson, M. A., Adedoyin, A. C., Brooks, M., Harmon, D. K., & Boamah, D. (2016). Hands up—Don't shoot: Police shooting of young Black males: Implications for social work and human services. *Journal of Human Behavior in the Social Environment, 26* (3–4), 254–266. https://doi.org/10.1080/10911359.2015.1125202

Morgaine, K., & Capous-Desyllas, M. J. (2014). *Anti-oppressive social work practice.* Newbury Park, CA: Sage Publishing.

National Association of Black Social Workers. (n.d.) *History.* https://www.nabsw.org/general/custom.asp?page=History

National Association of Social Workers. (2007). *Institutional racism & the social work profession: A call to action.* NASW President's Initiative, Weaving the Fabrics of Diversity, Presidential Task Force Subcommittee – Institutional Racism. https://www.socialworkers.org/LinkClick.aspx?fileticket=SWK1aR53FAk%3d&portalid=0

National Association of Social Workers. (2020a, July 14). *NASW seeks to dismantle racist policing.* https://www.socialworkers.org/News/News-Releases/ID/2205/NASW-Seeks-to-Dismantle-Racist-Policing

National Association of Social Workers. (2020b, August 21). *Social workers must help dismantle systems of oppression and fight racism within social work profession.* https://www.socialwor

kers.org/News/News-Releases/ID/2219/Social-Workers-Must-Help-Dismantle-Systems-of-Oppression-and-Fight-Racism-Within-Social-Work-Profession

Newman, Z. (2015). Hands up, don't shoot: Policing, fatal force, and equal protection in the age of colorblindness. *Hastings Constitutional Law Quarterly, 43*(1), 117–162. https://repository.uchastings.edu/hastings_constitutional_law_quaterly/vol43/iss1/4

Penketh, L., & Lavalette, M. (2014). Conclusion. In M. Lavalette & L. Penketh (Eds.), *Race, racism and social work: Contemporary issues and debates* (pp. 257–266). Bristol, UK: Polity Press.

Pon, G. (2009). Cultural competency as new racism: An ontology of forgetting. *Journal of Progressive Human Services, 20*(1), 59–71. https://doi.org/10.1080/10428230902871173

Reisch, M., & Andrews, J. (2002). *The road not taken: A history of radical social work in the United States.* New York, NY: Brunner-Routledge.

Ring, A. (2012). Provoking discomfort: A theoretical analysis of Racism at Columbia University school of social work. *Columbia Social Work Review, 6*, 5–17. https://doi.org/10.7916/D8PN9GG8

Rios, V. M., Prieto, G., & Ibarra, J. M. (2020). Mano suave-mano dura: Legitimacy policy and Latino stop-and-frisk. *American Sociological Review, 85*(1), 58–75. https://doi.org/10.1177/0003122419897348

Sakamoto, I. (2007). An anti-oppressive approach to cultural competence. *Canadian Social Work Review, 24(1),* 105–114.

Schroedel, J. R., & Chin, R. J. (2020). Whose lives matter: The media's failure to cover police use of lethal force against Native Americans. *Race and Justice, 10*(2), 150–175. https://doi.org/10.1177/2153368717734614

Schwartz, S. A. (2020). Police brutality and racism in America. *Explore*, 1–3. https://doi.org/10.1016/j.explore.2020.06.010

Singh, G. (2011, February 28). *Social work's anti-racist journey.* Community Care UK. https://www.communitycare.co.uk/2011/02/28/social-works-anti-racist-journey

Singh, G. (2014). Rethinking anti-racist social work in a neoliberal age. In M. Lavalette & L. Penketh (Eds.), *Race, racism and social work: Contemporary issues and debates* (pp. 17–31). Bristol, UK: Polity Press.

Smith, M. (2019, February 24). NYU social work school acknowledges 'institutional racism' after classroom episode. *Washington Post. Gale in Context: Opposing Viewpoints.* https://link-galecom.proxy2.cl.msu.edu/apps/doc/A575577273/OVIC?u=msu_main&sid=OVIC&xid=82c8b7a1.

Squire, S. (2020, July 12). Ida B. Wells, a writer who exposed the racist terror of lynching. *Socialist Worker*, Issue no. 2713. https://socialistworker.co.uk/art/50334/Ida+B+Wells%2C+a+writer+who+exposed+the+racist+terror+of_lynching

Trainin Blank, B. (n.d.). *Racism: The challenge for social workers.* https://www.socialworker.com/lecture-articles/ethics-articles-/Racism:_The_Challenge_for_Social_Workers/

Trolander, J. A. (1997). Fighting racism and sexism: The Council on Social Work Education. *The Social Service Review, 71*(1), 110–133. https://doi.org/10.1086/604233

Varghese, R. (2018). Teaching to transform? Addressing race and racism in the teachings of clinical social work practice. *Journal of Social Work Education, 52*, S134–S147. https://doi.org/10.1080/10437797.2016.1174646

Wells Barnett, I. B. (1901, May 16). Lynching and the excuse for it. *The Independent, 53*(2737), 1133–1136. https://hdl.handle.net/2027/coo.31924106546934?urlappend=%3Bseq=1157

From the archives: the Los Angeles riot study

Paul H. Stuart

The 1960s was a consequential decade for race relations in the United States. At mid-decade, it seemed that the long struggle to achieve the goal of racial integration would soon be achieved. Congress enacted a series of federal civil rights laws that ended de jure racial segregation and promised to achieve the major goals of the "second reconstruction" – the Civil Rights Acts of 1964 and 1968 and the Voting Rights Act of 1965. Yet less than a week after the signing of the Voting Rights Act, a riot broke out in South Los Angeles neighborhood of Watts, following the arrest of a 21-year-old African American driver, Marquette Frye, for suspected drunk driving. Like the Harlem Riots of 1964, which followed the police shooting of 15-year-old Jerome Powell, the Watts Riots differed from many earlier "race riots." While "race-related collective violence is a recurrent, periodic theme in American history," riots in the first half of the 20th century "were characterized by violent interracial clashes between blacks and whites, usually initiated by whites" while the disorders of the 1960s "featured clashes between blacks and law enforcement officials" (Lipsky & Olson, 1977, p. 37). Many argued that the riot, now called by some an uprising, reflected frustration at the continuing challenges of police brutality and segregation during a period of superficial progress. Years later, Frye, who had resisted arrest, told a reporter, "All I knew that day is that I was tired of being treated bad by a policeman" (Szymanski, 1990, para. 15).

Immediately after the riot, the Institute of Government and Public Affairs at the University of California, Los Angeles (UCLA) initiated the Los Angeles Riot Study (LARS). The study, funded by a grant from the Office of Economic Opportunity, was staffed by faculty members from a variety of social science disciplines. Nathan E. Cohen, a national social work leader who had joined the faculty of the UCLA School of Social Welfare in 1964, served as study coordinator. The Institute of Government and Public Affairs issued a preliminary report in 1967; the final report was issued five years after the riot (N. Cohen, 1970), after more than 300 other American cities had experienced serious riots (Lipsky & Olson, 1977, p. 10).

Politicians, social scientists, and social workers attempted to make sense of the riots during the late 1960s. Many of the riots were followed by official commissions, such as the McCone Commission, appointed by California's Governor, Edmund G. Brown, after the Los Angeles riot (Governor's Commission on the Los Angeles Riots [McCone Commission], 1965). President Lyndon B. Johnson appointed the Kerner Commission in July 1967, to "investigate the origins of the recent disorders in our cities [and] make recommendations–[to the President], to the Congress, to the State Governors, and to the mayors–for measures to prevent or contain such disasters in the future" (Johnson, 1967, para. 6). In their study of the official commissions of the 1960s, Lipsky and Olson (1977) conclude that riot commissions "initially function to provide evidence of action while postponing decisions" (p. 98).

The McCone Commission called for increased employment opportunities for African Americans and improvements in the educational system. However, it did not investigate allegations of widespread police brutality, though it recommended increasing police community relations efforts (Governor's Commission on the Los Angeles Riots [McCone Commission], 1965). The Kerner Commission went further; it warned of the increasing separation of the nation into "two societies, one black, one white – separate and unequal" and attributed the division to white racism (National Advisory Commission on Civil Disorders, 1968, p. 1). Although many believed the rioters were a small minority of the African American community, the LARS found that half or more of the residents of the riot area were participants in or "active observers" of the riot and that many residents of the riot area empathized with the protests expressed by the rioters (Cohen, 1967). The LARS social scientists interviewed African Americans and Whites who lived in or near the riot area, business owners, and a sample of Los Angeles County residents and were able to contrast White and African American opinions about the riots. LARS coordinator Nathan Cohen published a brief summary of the findings in *Social Work* in 1967; his article provides a convenient summary of the study's findings. The article concludes that the white community needed to be involved in solving the problems of inner-city Los Angeles. "The question is," Cohen (1967) wrote, "whether the nation ... will move to solve the racial problem within the spirit of its democratic heritage or whether it will resort primarily to power and force, risking change in the very nature of society" (p. 21).

The document

Nathan E. Cohen's article, "The Los Angeles Riot Study," appeared in the October 1967 issue of *Social Work* (vol. 12, no. 4). It is reprinted with the kind permission of Oxford University Press.

The Los Angeles Riot Study
By Nathan E. Cohen

Initiated immediately after the 1965 riot in Watts, the Los Angeles Riot Study undertook to survey samples of seven different basic populations: Negro, white, and Mexican-American curfew area residents, white residents of greater Los Angeles, arrested Negro rioters, social service workers, and merchants who incurred damage during the riot. Findings of the study indicate that popular beliefs about the riot (e.g., that it was caused by outside agitators) are erroneous, and may have significance for an understanding of the recent series of riots.

A growing body of myths has arisen about the riot that took place on August 11–15, 1965, in south central Los Angeles.[1] Statements being made about the riots that swept the country during this past summer are similar to those made immediately after the events in Watts. These center around the effort to distinguish between the "good" Negro and the "bad" Negro. A correlate is the belief that the riots are the work of outside agitators, "riffraff," or the "mad dog" element of Negroes. A guessing game follows: What is the percentage of "bad" Negroes in the population? (Two to 5% seems to be a popular figure.) All of this serves to divert attention from the social ills responsible for the riots, leading to the rationalization that they can be dealt with by a better use of police power.

Data gathered by a group of social scientists at the Institute of Government and Public Affairs, University of California, Los Angeles, in a two-year study of the Watts riot indicate that popular beliefs held about the riot are erroneous.[2] Some of the findings of this study may contribute to a better understanding of the recent series of riots.

The Los Angeles Riot Study (LARS) was initiated immediately after the 1965 Los Angeles riot. During the five months following the riot a total of 2,070 personal interviews were collected in a survey that sampled seven basic populations: (1) Negro curfew area residents, (2) arrested Negro rioters, (S) white residents of greater Los Angeles, (4) white curfew area residents, (5) Mexican-American curfew area residents, (6) social service workers, and (7) merchants who incurred damage during the riot. Interviews were about two hours in length and the schedule covered questions of attitude toward the riot, activity in the riot, general social and political attitudes, and background information. Interviewers were selected from the area.

The sample of Negro curfew area residents was a random one, stratified by age, sex, and income. It may be helpful to describe the characteristics of this group:

1. The majority spent their childhood in the South.

2. Over 60% grew up in urban areas (suburb, large or medium-sized city).

3. About 60% had lived in Los Angeles ten years or longer at the time of the riot.

4. Over 50% had completed high school.

5. If the concept of the "job ceiling" is applied to refer to those positions above the level of semiskilled, only about 25 per-cent of the males and 18% of the females in the sample are above this level.

6. Seventy-two percent of the males and 35% of the females in the sample are employed. The percentage of unemployment is much higher for the females (42%) than for the males (15%).

Major findings

In regard to participation in the riot, the LARS study suggests these:

1. Up to 15% of the Negro adult population, or about 22,000 persons, were active at some point during the rioting, and in more than a "spectator" role.

2. An additional 35 or 40% of the Negro adult population, or at least an additional 51,000 persons, were active spectators to the disturbance.

3. Young people were much more active than older people.

4. Men were more active than women, but young women were more active than middle-aged or older men.

5. Support for the riot was as great among relatively well0educated and economically advantaged persons as among the poorly educated and economically disadvantaged in the curfew areas.

6. Support for the riot was as great among relatively long-time residents of south central Los Angeles as it was among the more recent migrants from the South. Furthermore, the data indicate that the majority of people in south central Los Angeles are long-time residents, thus dispelling the belief that the riot was the product of a recent influx of migrants from the South.

Perhaps as important as the proportion of persons involved in the riot is the extent to which residents of the community gave approval to it:

1. About 34% of the sample were somewhat or very favorable toward it.

2. While the majority expressed disapproval of the violence and destruction, this was often coupled with an expression of empathy with the motives of those who participated, or a sense of pride that the Negro has brought worldwide attention to his problem.

Another important measure of attitude is the assessment of the residents of the community of the consequences of the riot for the Negro cause and for relations with white persons. Considerable optimism was shown over the results of the riot

1. Thirty-eight percent of the population in the curfew area felt that the riot would help the Negro cause. Only about 20% felt that it would hurt the cause. A study of the white population in the Los Angeles metropolitan area was in sharp contrast. Seventy-four percent believed the riot would hurt the cause of the Negro.

2. Only 23% of the population in the curfew area felt that the riot increased the gap between the races, as contrasted with 71% of the white population.

3. Fifty-one percent of the population in the curfew area saw the whites as now being more sympathetic because of the riot as against 32% of the whites.

Social ills in Watts

Preriot conditions in Watts reflect the entire gamut of social problems in the slum ghetto. There were the usual deficits in employment, housing, education, and health and welfare services. For example, there were twelve social agencies prior to 1964 in Watts, eleven new ones were started between 1964 and 1965, and nineteen additional ones were instituted after the riot. Those launched in 1964 were primarily related to the poverty program but their effectiveness was limited by a running battle in the community between city hall and the voluntary agencies as to where the power was to be located.

In addition, the following factors were found to be characteristic of the social service delivery system in Watts:

1. Only half of the agencies had provisions for emergency service in an area that has high requirements for such service.

2. The requirements of highly specialized agencies governing the conditions under which service could be obtained made it extremely difficult for those most in need to be eligible.

3. Most of the new poverty program agencies had no waiting lists for service but the agencies offering highly skilled professional services in health, mental health, and family services did have them.

4. Only a small minority of agencies had representatives of the client population on their policy-making boards.

In general, the majority of agencies did seem to block access to their services with excessive intake demands and long waiting lists. However, there was limited case-finding or reaching out for people who could not connect without some additional help. If the individual or family did not have the strength to go to the agency and stay there, he went unserved. The highest level of expertise was not frequently available to the low-income resident of Watts even when the agency was located in the areas. It was felt that this may lead to an increased sense of relative deprivation, which is so often the seed of violence.

The grievances of the people in Watts were numerous. These ran the gamut of the practices of merchants operating in the community, various types of discrimination, and alleged forms of mistreatment by the police. Analysis of the data suggests this:

1. When asked to state their biggest gripe, 33% cited poor neighborhood conditions, 14% mistreatment by whites, and 13% economic conditions. Only 21% had no specific complaints.

2. When asked specifically about exploitive practices by merchants, approximately one-third claimed to have encountered "frequently" the experience of being overcharged and sold inferior goods.

3. When asked about job discrimination, 54% of the males and 33% of the females mentioned that they personally had experienced it.

4. Males were also more likely to report discrimination in housing, practices by landlords, and schools. Thirty-four percent of the males stated that they had experienced discrimination in housing.

"Police brutality" is frequently mentioned as a major factor in the Los Angeles riot. An analysis of the data indicates that well above a majority of both sexes believe that most forms of police malpractice – including the more violent such as use of unnecessary force in arrests, beating up people in custody, and searching homes unnecessarily – occur in this community. Few of the respondents, however, have experienced this. When it comes to such malpractice as insulting comments, rousting or frisking individuals unnecessarily, and stopping or searching cars without cause, approximately one-third of the males in the sample reported one or more such occurrences, and about 50% reported that they had seen it happen. Less than 15% of the females reported direct experience, but about 30% reported seeing it happen.

Another important factor in assessing the Los Angeles riot is the extent of social contact of Negroes in the curfew area with whites, and their feelings about whites. The data suggest the following:

1. Approximately half of the sample (45% of the males and 42% of the females) reported social contact with whites.

2. Among both sexes the overwhelming majority seemed to have little objection to white interaction of whatever intimacy.

BEYOND LIP SERVICE

3. About 90% of both sexes stated that they would prefer working in a racially mixed group.

4. Approximately 18% of the males and 15% of the females said they did not trust any white person. Over 70% of both sexes stated they could trust some, and approximately 9% said they could trust most.

White reactions

The white community can be both a help and a barrier in solving the racial problem. Their perceptions and deeds are an integral part of understanding the social fabric within which the riot took place. The findings from the white reaction study of LARS provide the following information:

1. In characterizing the events of August 11–15, their causes and purpose, about a third of the white respondents showed some sympathy toward the disturbance.

2. Nineteen percent stated that it helped and 74% said it hurt the Negro cause.

3. Seventy-three percent stated that it had increased and 13% that it had decreased the gap between the races.

4. Thirty-two percent of the sample thought whites were more sympathetic since the riot and 37% thought they were less sympathetic.

5. Sixty-six percent thought the authorities handled the riot well, 31% badly.

6. Over half the whites felt some or a great deal of fear.

7. Nearly one-third considered using firearms, over one-half approved of buying guns, and some 12% either bought or already had firearms.

8. Roughly one-third of the whites had an exaggerated idea of the size of the disturbance and the number of Negroes supporting it (even after three months of factual reports on the riot).

9. Some 20% felt that the best way to prevent further riots was to take punitive or restrictive action of one form or another.

10. On measures of stereotypes and beliefs about racial differences, social distance questions, attitudes of dislike and distrust of Negroes, and attitudes about Negro efforts to improve their position through social action the findings were as follows:

a. The least amount of antagonism is found with regard to stereotypes, racial beliefs, and impersonal social relations.

b. Most antagonism is in the areas of social action programs and close social relationships.

The most important factor in determining the reaction of whites to the disturbance appears to be their more basic attitudes toward Negroes. Respondents who are relatively antagonistic toward Negroes tend to view the riot as the result of outside "agitation," to believe the riot hurt the

Negro's cause, and to suggest punitive solutions to the problem. Conversely, respondents who are tolerant in their general attitudes toward Negroes tend to see the causes of the riot in such sources as white prejudice and discrimination against Negroes or lack of employment and educational opportunities, are more likely to believe the riot helped the Negro's cause, and are more likely to suggest ameliorative solutions to the problem, such as full civil rights for Negroes and increased educational and economic opportunities.

Proress since the riot

Several key issues emerging from these findings warrant further exploration. The Negro community was ambivalent toward the riot itself, but a majority saw it as bringing positive results. The riot was viewed as a way of bringing their plight to the attention of the white community, with the assumption that if the whites knew the real conditions existing in Watts they would act rationally and in good American tradition take the appropriate steps to reform the situation. For the Negro the riot might help to hasten the creation of jobs and general improvement of the neighborhood and its institutions dealing with education, welfare, social control, health, recreation, housing, transportation, and consumer malpractices. We must ask ourselves honestly whether his has happened.

It is not enough to be able to state that some progress has been made. Gradual change in a period crying for rapid change is not enough. Statistics can show that there have been some small increases in employment and some narrowing of the economic gap between the white and the Negro. There is the danger, however, of falling into the trap of the scientist who drowned in the river because he was informed that its average depth was four feet.

Since the Los Angeles riot, white political and civic leaders have apparently become more responsive to Negro demands. To this point, such responsiveness is more verbal and visible than it is substantive: the degree of policy change that can be observed is minimal; there is furthermore a tendency within the political party system for a Democratic political leadership to take the Negro as a traditional democrat "given" and contrariwise for Republican Party leaders to write off the Negro vote.

The McCone Commission Report recommendations represent a maximum program to most whites, including most white leaders, but only a minimum and largely symbolic program not only to the Negro leadership, but to Negroes in general. The very nature of the political structure is producing barriers to the accomplishment of even these "minimal" recommendations.

The division of authority and function between city and county and also between state and federal levels of government makes it difficult to pursue even a single goal (such as housing). The weak mayor-council tradition and the proliferation of independent boards and commissions of the city (e.g., the "civilian" police commission) also inhibit effective Negro political action.

Nonpartisan elections and, in the case of the Los Angeles Unified School Board, at-large districts also operate to discount the numerical significance of Negro electoral power.

Much of the expansion of resources has come from the federal government. There has been growing uncertainty as to the availability of funds and many programs are never sure about their survival. Summer programs tend to be funded at the beginning of the summer and even in mid-summer rather than a year in advance so that appropriate plans can be made. There is also evidence of a growing congressional resistance to legislation dealing with the problems of the slum ghettos. Crucial programs such as model cities, rent supplements, aid to education, the community action program of the Office of Economic Opportunity, and rat control have become political footballs. More basic programs such as a massive public works project, guaranteed jobs, encouragement of the private sector to participate in slum problems through tax incentives, and a guaranteed annual income have not reached the drawing board.

Polarization of Negro groupings

A second key consideration is the growing polarization of three groupings in the Negro community, namely, the "traditionalists," the "militants," and the "survivalists." The Administration's policies and programs vis-à-vis the Negro problem have tended more to stress the traditional model of individual success than to view the problems of the group as a whole. As a result, a pattern has been encouraged in the Negro community that places a premium on individual mobility rather than collective concern. The Negro community has witnessed the emergence of the "Talented Tenth" projected by W. E. B. DuBois, but find that this group, which has grown beyond the 10% envisioned, has tended to operate in the more traditional ways and has lost touch with the plight of the 35–40% of the Negro population whose pervasive concern is not status frustration, but rather economic frustration.[3] The latter group can best be characterized as victims of disease, desperation, joblessness, and hopelessness. They are highly visible on the welfare rolls and if employed tend to be underemployed. They contribute heavily to the poverty statistics. Their primary concern is survival.

Between these two groups – the traditionalists and the survivalists – is a growing group of the Negro population who are questioning the strategy of the traditionalists and the programs of the government. These militants are seeking new solutions. They vary in their philosophy but have as a common denominator the belief that individual mobility is not the answer and that only through collective concern can the Negro solve his problems. Included in this group is a new urban Negro who is least representative of yesterday's Negro. The core of this group are educated, tend to come from educated families, are less religious, and do not identify themselves as lower class. They are making strong efforts to build a sense of pride in their color and to rebuild a sense of ethnicity. For them the white man has not yet demonstrated that he is to be trusted.

The emergence of the militants comes through sharply in the LARS study around questions determining opinions toward militant organizations. Those who approved of the militant organizations were classified as militants, those who disapproved were classified as conservatives, and those who were unfamiliar or indifferent to militant organizations were classified as uninvolved. An analysis of the data around this tripartite typology suggests this:

1. Each group was represented by approximately equal thirds of the population. (Militants, approximately 30%; conservatives, approximately 35%; and the uninvolved, approximately 35%.)

2. There were no marked differences between the groups on such factors as birthplace, sex, education, length of residence in Los Angeles, political party, or declared social class.

3. One background characteristic that was significantly different is employment. More of the militants (70%) and the conservatives (63%) are employed that the uninvolved (55%). Thus the militant Negro is as likely as any other Negro to be a job holder.

In the area of attitudes there are several significant differences among the three groups:

1. Militants are significantly less favorable to the news media (radio, television, newspapers) than the conservatives and tend to view them as unfair in their portrayal of the Negro and his problems. The uninvolved tend to fall about midway between the militants and the conservatives in their evaluation of news media.

2. Political institutions (state legislature, city council, and the like) were less favorably evaluated by the militants than by the conservatives, the uninvolved again falling midway between the two.

3. Political figures – local, state, and national – were relatively devalued by the militants compared to the conservatives, the uninvolved again falling between.

4. Civil rights organizations were valued highly by all groups, but the group least favorable toward any organizations was the uninvolved. The militants lent strongest approval to the more militant organizations, but in general they were not different from the conservatives in their clear approval of any civil rights organization.

Characteristics of militants

In view of the recent explosion of riots and the ascendancy of the militant or activist ideology it may be helpful to outline their characteristics in greater detail. The profile that emerges from the findings of the study suggests the following: The militants were more action oriented than the conservatives, were significantly more willing to engage in civil rights demonstrations, significantly more active in demonstrations prior to the riot, more often approached by civil rights organizations, and were more sophisticated and active in traditional political activity (voting and other political behavior).

The militant claimed greater degrees of and more extensive varieties of grievances than the conservatives. He saw significantly more police brutality in all forms from insults to physical assault. He believed to a greater extent than the conservatives that merchants victimized Negroes and he saw greater degrees of discrimination in schools, jobs, housing, and the like than his conservative counterpart.

The militant is both angry and active and his message backs up his feelings and action. When asked whether the events of August constituted a riot or a revolt, he claimed significantly more often than the conservative that they were a revolt. The militant gave uniformly greater approval to the Los Angeles riot and expressed greater belief that the riot would have positive outcomes for Negroes. He also declared a greater likelihood of a recurrence of rioting in Los Angeles, and selected violence significantly more frequently than the conservative as the most effective method for the Negro to gain equality.

The militants are no longer impressed with the upward mobility of the traditionalists and tend to regard them with suspicion and as "Uncle Toms." They are competing with the traditionalists for the leadership role in delivering the survivalists out of the wilderness. To do this they realize that they must develop economic and political power, to which they now refer as Black Power.

The traditionalists, with their emphasis on status frustration, can be more oriented to the future than the survivalists, whose priority concern is economic frustration. The militant, with his focus on both status and economic frustration, is becoming more attractive to the survivalist. For those whose plight and condition make them oriented to the present, the militant offers the most attractive plan, pointing out as he does that the Negro has gained little through the slow legislative processes and the results will come more immediately if he takes matters into his own hands. To the survivalist whose life has not been materially changed by conventional civil rights activities and by an expansion of services, many of which are oriented to the future, and who daily sees little indication of a real interest on the part of the white community in changing his condition, the interpretation of their plight by the militants and the call to action become exceedingly attractive.

The traditionalists still have the primary access to the Administration and to the white Establishment. They are still being relied on to deliver the Negro com unity politically and to keep the lid on the pressure cooker of mounting action. They are having growing difficulty, however, in maintaining their leadership, which is dependent on the ability of the administration to deliver on a much larger scale than at present the essential policies and programs that deal with economic frustration. As stated by Roy Wilkins:

> The reality is that all levels of government, local, state, and federal, have bolstered the "wreck 'em" theory of Negro separatist politics and the brinksmanship of Negro crusaders by their mincing politics and partisan political maneuvers.[4]

The reaction of the white community to the riot would indicate that there is a hardening of their position on race relations, a polarization of their attitudes into a potential white backlash, and an increased use of force.

In regard to the handling of the riot, 64% of the population in the curfew area thought it was handled badly and only 28% thought it was handled well. In the white community 66% saw it as handled well and 31% as handled poorly. This "worries" the traditionalists in their effort to obtain gains through the usual legislative and court processes. The militants, however, would argue that the whites are merely using the riots as a rationalization to avoid doing what they had not planned to do in the first place. They feel that it is more important to keep before the survivalists and atmosphere of the white as the enemy, and before the whites a fear of a growing militant group who will stop at nothing to attain their goal. This stance against an outside enemy, they feel, will help to build a unity among Negroes and will strengthen their position to demand more for their people.

Essentially, the militants are committed to a strategy of disrupting the system as a means of gaining greater bargaining power for helping the Negro move more rapidly into the economic and political streams. The social stream – integration – is no longer the primary goal. Integration becomes an individual rather than a group goal. What they are seeking is the right of any individual to have a choice. This is a long-range concern, however, and the power necessary to achieve it can be found through greater strength in the political and economic arenas. This in turn necessitates, at this time, building a greater sense of identity, unity, and nationalist spirit.

The method of the militants is to create fear and hostility in the white community. The white community's stance traditionally has been to ask the Negro to prove himself if he is to gain access to society. They have controlled the timetable by controlling the avenues of opportunity. The Negroes have witnessed the whites' ambivalence between encouraging their progress and erecting barriers to achieving their share of the American Dream. It is difficult of the whites to accept the Negroes' contention that what they are asking for is their rights as citizens and not for something that belongs exclusively to the whites, to be doled out to Negroes as the whites think they are ready for it. For the Negro this smacks of colonialism, a system they have seen go down to defeat elsewhere in recent years.

Need for comprehensive approach

What is needed is a comprehensive approach to the racial problem that reflects a knowledge of the differential aspects of the three groupings described earlier, their interrelationships, and the core of their common concerns as well as their differences. This will necessitate dialogue with representation from all three groups. The white community's hostility toward the militants should not blind them to the growing role or this group in the Negro community. The question of jobs should be first on the agenda. Also high on the agenda should be issues such as poor neighborhood conditions, discriminatory practices, and social control malpractices. Also essential are the role and responsibility of the larger context within which the Negro community operates, namely, the white community. The white community is both helper and barrier to the solution of the problems. The Negro community is looking for tangible evidence that the nation has not lost its sense of commitment to what they had come to believe was being regarded as the major problem of our times. They are pondering the various solutions being debated within their own ranks. Their direction will be affected markedly by the economic, political, and social climate. If, for example, they discern a regressive climate that stresses increased police power as the answer – similar to the back-to-the-woodshed theory in delinquency – rather that the view expressed by former Attorney General Nicholas Katzenbach (namely, that the most dangerous agitators in the ghettos are disease and desperation, joblessness and hopelessness), then the program of the extreme militants will of necessity find favor.

The question is whether the nation, emerging out of its trauma of the past summer, will move to solve the racial problem within the spirit of its democratic heritage or whether it will resort primarily to power and force, risking change in the very nature of society. It is imperative that in forging next steps all the facts and knowledge available be utilized so that decisions and plans are both wise and just. Order must be maintained, but not as a substitute for dealing with the urban and racial condition. The solution is neither simple nor without massive costs. It demands the full co-operation and sacrifice of the total community. The problem lies with human beings and cries for a human answer. It is inhuman to seek solutions through a desire for partisan political gains. It is blind and unjust to seek them through fear and prejudice. What is at stake is more than the plight of the Negro. It is the future of the democratic way of life and of humanity.

Notes

1. Although the riot spread beyond its initial focal point, Watts, for brevity the term Watts will be used here to refer to the entire curfew area.
2. Members of the research staff, in addition to the author, were Jerome Cohen, Eugene L. Loren, Richard T. Morris, Vincent Jeffries, Raymond J. Murphy, James Watson, Walter J. Raine, Harry M. Scoble, David O. Sears, Thomas M. Tomlinson, and Diana TenHouten.
3. DuBois' thesis was that if the upper 10% of the Negro group could receive college education, as contrasted with Booker T. Washington's emphasis on elementary and vocational training, they would serve as a leadership group to help pull up the masses.
4. *Los Angeles Times*, January 2, 1967, Part II-5.

Afterword

Much of the nation's response to the problems of urban unrest involved increasing "power and force" to suppress rioting in spite of the warnings of Cohen and others. In 1967, Cohen testified before the Senate Judiciary Committee to oppose a bill "that would make interstate travel to incite a riot a federal crime" (Burke, 1967, August 22, p. 9). The bill had been passed by the House of Representatives, and liberals on the Judiciary Committee invited Cohen to testify. Drawing on the LARS findings, Cohen argued that a punitive response to urban disorder would increase African American sympathy for the rioters:

> I think there is ... empathy around the fact that Negroes are finally showing that they would not take it, that they are expressing a set of feelings that many of these people have themselves, and there is some feeling of pride. I think it is more of this point of view that is being expressed. My concern is that if we do go regressive, more punitive, we are going to feed this view even more (Anti-Riot Bill, 1967, p. 608)

The anti-rioting bill was not passed by the Senate in 1967, but was enacted as the Anti-Riot Act, Title X of the 1968 Civil Rights Act. The inclusion of the Anti-Riot Act was a compromise designed to secure conservative support for the larger act, which prohibited housing discrimination (Zalman, 1975). The Anti-Riot Act has been used infrequently; the best-known defendants were the Chicago seven, who were charged with conspiring to disrupt the 1968 Democratic Convention in Chicago (Ragsdale, 2008). More recently, the law has been used against neo-Nazis and, during the Trump administration, against Black Lives Matter protestors (Reilly, 2020, September 24).

The inclusion of the Anti-Riot Act in the last major civil rights statute of Lyndon Johnson's administration was ironic and prophetic. Earlier in 1968, the Kerner Commission had warned of the increasing separation of the nation into "two societies, one black, one white – separate and unequal" (National Advisory Commission on Civil Disorders, 1968, p. 1). While the Kerner Commission attributed the divisions to White racism, critics charged that the commission had neglected to emphasize the power differential between Whites and Blacks, especially economic inequality (Gillon, 2018). But many Whites were hostile to the Kerner Commission Report, particularly what they saw as its failure to assign blame to the rioters. Richard Nixon, who had "reinvented himself as a centrist and racial moderate" after Barry Goldwater's defeat in the 1964 Presidential election, criticized the report and the Johnson administration's response to the riots (Gillon, 2018, p. 280). Nixon portrayed himself as a defender of law and order against the chaos brought on by the riots.

A quarter century after the Watts Riots, the members of the Kerner Commission presented a bleak assessment of the situation of poor urban African Americans. Commission member John Lindsey wrote in 1987 that the commission should have emphasized "the growing development in the United States of an economically depressed underclass" (Gillon, 2018, p. 305). "The conditions now, in my view, are unquestionably worse in the inner cities" than they had been in the 1960s, Kerner Commission executive director David Ginsburg observed in 1992 (Gillon, 2018, p. 304). A half century after the Watts Riots, the UCLA Luskin School of Public Affairs found that there had been little progress since the 1960s; the earnings gap between workers in South Los Angeles and in Los Angeles County as a whole had widened, fewer South L.A. residents owned their homes, and public schools remained "separate and unequal" (Ong, Comandon, Cheng, & González, 2018, p. 29).

Educated as a psychologist, Nathan E. Cohen decided to leave experimental psychology and pursue social justice after seeing Mussolini's Black Shirts marching below his window during a fellowship in Italy in the 1930s (Saxon, 2001). He worked for a number of private agencies and joined the faculty of the New York School of Social Work. He served as the first president of the National Association of Social Workers from 1955 to 1957. Cohen later served as Dean of the School of Applied Social Sciences at Western Reserve University He joined the UCLA faculty in 1964 and retired in 1977. Nathan E. Cohen died in 2001; obituaries appeared in the *Los Angeles Times* (Woo, 2001, February 3) and the *New York Times* (Saxon, 2001).

For further reading. There is a rich literature on the urban civil disorders of the 1960s. Lipsky and Olson (1977) provides an analysis of the official commissions that investigated the 1960s urban civil disorders, including the McCone Commission (Governor's Commission on the Los Angeles Riots [McCone Commission], 1965) and the Kerner Commission (National Advisory Commission on Civil Disorders, 1968). The report of the UCLA Los Angeles Riot Study (N. Cohen, 1970) can supplementand correct many of the McCone Commission's findings. Among many other secondary accounts, Carter (2009)and Gillon (2018)provide helpful accounts of the Johnson Administration's response to urban unrest in the 1960s and the origins and results of the Kerner Commission. Ong et al. (2018)provide an assessment of changes in South Los Angeles since the Los Angeles Riot of 1965. A special issue of *RSF: The Russell Sage Foundation Journal of the Social Sciences* (Gooden & Myers, 2018) assesses the Kerner Report and its impact on African American neighborhoods.

Disclosure statement

No potential conflict of interest was reported by the author(s).

References

Bill, A.-R. (1967). *Hearings before the United States Senate Committee on the Judiciary, Ninetieth Congress, first session.* U.S. Government Printing Office. https://babel.hathitrust.org/cgi/pt?id=umn.31951d021723864&view=1up&seq=9&skin=2021

Burke, V. J. (1967, August 22). Expert on Watts warns of "pride in aggression": More police power won't remove riot causes, UCLA professor tells Senators. *The Los Angeles Times*, 9. https://www.proquest.com/docview/155831555/248FFF6938D34DA3PQ/1?accountid=10901

Carter, D. C. (2009). *The Music has gone out of the Movement: Civil Rights and the Johnson Administration, 1965-1968.* University of North Carolina Press.

Cohen, N. E. (1967). The Los Angeles riot study. *Social Work, 12*(4), 14–21. https://www.jstor.org/stable/23710409

Cohen, N. (1970). *The Los Angeles riots: A socio-psychological study.* Praeger. https://archive.org/details/losangelesriotss0000unse/page/n9/mode/2up?view=theater

Gilllon, S. M. (2018). *Separate and Unequal: The Kerner Commission and the Unraveling of American Liberalism.* Basic Books.

Gooden, S. T., and Myers, S. L., Jr., eds. (2018). The fiftieth anniversary of the Kerner Commission report [special issue]. *RSF: The Russell Sage Foundation Journal of the Social Sciences, 4*(6), 12–41. https://www.rsfjournal.org/content/4/6

Governor's Commission on the Los Angeles Riots [McCone Commission] (1965). Violence in the city: An end or a beginning? https://www.lc.edu/uploadedFiles/Pages/Services/Reid_Memorial_Library/McCone%20Commission%20Report%20Violence%20in%20the%20City%20Watts%20Neighborhood.pdf

Johnson, L. B. (1967). The President's Address to the Nation on Civil Disorders, July 27, 1967. The President's Address to the Nation on Civil Disorders. https://www.presidency.ucsb.edu/documents/the-presidents-address-the-nation-civil-disorders.

Lipsky, M., & Olson, D. J. (1977). *Commission politics: The processing of racial crisis in America.* Transaction Books. https://archive.org/details/commissionpoliti0000lips/page/n3/mode/2up

National Advisory Commission on Civil Disorders [Kerner Commission] (1968). Report. Washington, D. C: U.S. Government Printing Office. Available at https://catalog.hathitrust.org/Record/000339500

Ong, P. M., Comandon, A., Cheng, A., & González, S. R. (2018). South Los Angeles since the Sixties: Half a Century of Progress? Center for Neighborhood Knowledge, University of California, Los Angeles. https://knowledge.luskin.ucla.edu/about/

Ragsdale, B. A. (2008). *The Chicago Seven: 1960s radicalism in the federal courts.* Federal Judicial Center. https://www.fjc.gov/sites/default/files/trials/chicago7.pdf

Reilly, R. J. (2020, September 24). How segregationists rushed through the 1968 rioting laws DOJ is using in 2020. *Huffington Post.* https://www.huffpost.com/entry/anti-rioting-act-civil-disorder-law-doj-barr-trump-consitutional_n_5f6a012cc5b655acbc701ca2

Saxon, W. (2001, February 13). Nathan Cohen, 91; helped reshape social work. *New York Times*, Section B, p. 8.

Szymanski, M. (1990, August 5). How legacy of the Watts riot consumed, ruined man's life. Orlando. *Sentinel.* https://www.orlandosentinel.com/news/os-xpm-1990-08-05-9008031131-story.html

Woo, E. (2001, February 3). Obituaries: Nathan Cohen; Expert broadened social work's focus. *The Los Angeles Times, B6.* https://www.proquest.com/docview/421647715/fulltext/1B35367647140F5PQ/1?accountid=10901

Zalman, M. (1975). The Federal Anti-Riot Act and political crime: The need for criminal law theory. *Villanova Law Review, 20*(5–6), 897–937. https://digitalcommons.law.villanova.edu/cgi/viewcontent.cgi?article=2069&context=vlr

Beyond community policing: centering community development in efforts to improve safety in Latinx immigrant communities

Willow Lung-Amam, Nohely Alvarez, and Rodney Green

ABSTRACT
Recent uprisings have led to calls to defund police and invest in Black and Brown communities. This article explores the lessons learned about community safety from a four-year effort to reduce crime and improve safety in a predominately Latinx suburb of Washington, DC. It shows that programs that invested in building trust and rapport between police and community had little impact. Alternatively, efforts that built community, resourced and engaged residents, and invested in neighborhood infrastructure were more effective. The case highlights the critical role of community-based organizations in helping residents imagine and execute programs that improve community safety without relying on police.

One's zip code is often a primary indicator of one's access to opportunity. Decades of policies that segregated, contained, underinvested in, and exploited Black and Brown neighborhoods have left many with high poverty rates, failing healthcare systems, underfunded schools, crumbling infrastructure, and a lack of employment opportunities – all of which contribute to high crime rates and public safety concerns (Sampson & Loeffler, 2010). Yet the government's spatial fix to address crime in these neighborhoods has not often addressed these underlying conditions; it has instead intensely policed them.

Policing, however, rarely makes Black and Brown communities feel or objectively become safer (Alexander, 2011). Instead, excessive fines and fees, racially disparate sentencing, and mass incarceration often leave communities of color further behind, hampering the educational and employment opportunities for incarcerated and formerly incarcerated individuals and their families. Policing disrupts entire neighborhoods. It undermines public confidence and restrains human capacities and assets that contribute to economic growth and disrupts vital social networks and capital development (Gilmore, 2007; Simpson et al., 2020). In Latinx neighborhoods, federal and local anti-immigrant policing further restrains and blocks improvement in the capacities of individuals and communities.

Community policing is often proposed as a solution to reduce crime and increase residents' sense of safety by building trust with police and communities (Skogan, 2006; Stein & Griffith, 2015). In many Black and Brown neighborhoods, however, residents often perceive the mere presence of police as putting them more at risk, increasing their likelihood of becoming victims of police violence, and ending up in the criminal justice system, deported, or dead (Chaney & Robertson, 2013). A popular federal community policing model is the Community-Based Crime Reduction (CBCR) program supported by the U.S. Department of Justice (DOJ). This program seeks to build partnerships between police and communities in high-poverty, disadvantaged neighborhoods to develop data-driven strategies targeting "hot spots" of criminal activity (Hipple & Saunders, 2020).

Based on our engagement as researchers in a four-year CBCR planning and implementation project in a predominantly Latinx inner-ring suburb in the Washington, DC metropolitan area, we explore the project's outcomes in reducing crime and increasing residents' sense of safety. Overall, the project did not show significant drops in crime or changes in residents' sense of safety during the two years of project implementation. Further, the project's community policing efforts that sought to build better community-police relations and equip police with tools to better understand and communicate with residents showed limited positive outcomes. In some cases, they decreased or deterred resident participation. Alternatively, efforts led by residents and focused on neighborhood investments, including infrastructure improvements, resident education, resource access, and capacity and community-building had more positive and potentially long-lasting results. This case highlights the critical role of community-based organizations in helping residents imagine and execute programs that improve community safety without relying solely or even primarily on police.

Community policing and safety in immigrant neighborhoods

Despite numerous studies showing the immigrants are less likely than native-born residents to engage in crime, Latinx immigrant neighborhoods are often the subject of hyper-surveillance, over-policing, and racialized policing (Garcia-Hallett et al., 2020; Martinez, 2002; Saint-Fort et al., 2012; Sampson & Loeffler, 2010). These practices are not only prevalent in cities, but also in suburbs where most new immigrants live (Roth & Grace, 2018).

In many Black and Brown neighborhoods, community policing programs have been adopted to engage residents in creating strategies with police to address crime and safety issues (Skogan, 2006). Many Latinx immigrant neighborhoods, however, face myriad challenges that hamper community policing efforts. Residents often distrust police and fear retaliation from neighbors and police, reducing the likelihood of their reporting crime and working with police to solve crimes (Saint-Fort et al., 2012). They also are often uncomfortable with legal systems because of language barriers, experiences in their countries of origin, or their legal status (Garcia-Hallett et al., 2020; Roth & Grace, 2018). Local and federal anti-immigrant programs, such as Secure Communities and Section 287(g) of the Immigration and Nationality Act, also undermine effective community policing and other public safety initiatives by increasing fear and decreasing engagement among immigrants, both documented and undocumented (Xie & Baumer, 2019).

The role of police in practice, however, often goes well beyond solving or addressing crime. Given a lack of municipal funding for community development programs, police often undertake the roles of community mental health practitioners and social workers. A lack of training for police in these areas and their implicit biases often lead them to have higher perceptions of crime and disorder in low-income communities of color than residents (Skogan, 2006). In Latinx immigrant communities, residents are more inclined to work with police on community safety efforts when they partner with trusted local nonprofits and community-based institutions and support local activities (Garcia-Hallett et al., 2020).

Community development efforts that decenter policing and promote a neighborhood's social assets demonstrate the importance of leveraging resident and local stakeholder voices in creating safe communities (Lane & Henry, 2004). Robust investments in critical programs such as mental health, education, and job training while prioritizing community voice and leadership has increased safety in many neighborhoods (Lane & Henry, 2004; Saint-Fort et al., 2012). However, both the literature on community policing and effective community development strategies to increase safety have had a limited focus on Latinx immigrant neighborhoods, particularly those in suburbia – the focus of this case study.

Crime and safety in a Latinx immigrant suburb

Langley Park is an unincorporated area of Prince George's County that occupies less than a square mile near Washington, DC's northeast border. Built out as a post-World War II suburb for the White working-class, by the 1980s immigrants from Latin America and the Caribbean, Southeast Asia, and Africa began arriving, as White flight took hold (Naughton, 1991). Today, Langley Park is a predominantly Latinx immigrant suburb. In 2018, 83% of its more than 19,000 residents were Latinx and 12% were Black.[1] Over half (60%) were immigrants, with 82% of those emigrating from Central America, largely Guatemala and El Salvador. Among the neighborhood's Black population, 42% are immigrants, mainly from the Caribbean and Sub-Saharan Africa. The neighborhood is widely considered the heart of the Latinx community in the DC metro area, with one of the largest populations of Latinx and immigrants in Maryland, including many undocumented residents (Lung-Amam et al., 2019). In contrast, only one in five county residents and only 11% of the Prince George's County Police Department (PGPD) officers are Latinx.

The neighborhood faces challenges related to poverty, health care, education, and employment. Langley Park's median household income of $61,895 is 24% lower than that of Prince George's County. One in five residents lives below the poverty line. Over half lack access to health insurance. Only 38% of adults over 25 have a high school degree or higher. Adults often work in the construction industry with low wages, unstable employment, and few benefits. The neighborhood's official unemployment rate is 5.4% compared to 3.8% statewide.

Langley Park is nonetheless a close-knit community with strong social capital and a network of neighborhood-serving small businesses and organizations. In a 2019 CBCR community survey, 71% of respondents felt like they belong in the neighborhood and 65% regularly talked with neighbors. The neighborhood also has many churches, nonprofits, and immigrant-serving small businesses where residents regularly gather. CASA, the Mid-Atlantic's largest immigrant rights organization, is a longstanding community organization that runs a community development program in the neighborhood and offers many popular health, legal, social, education, and employment services to residents.

Community policing interventions

CASA applied for and won a CBCR implementation grant in 2018 that built on their 2016 CBCR planning grant and other efforts to address ongoing public safety initiatives in Langley Park. Prince George's County had previously designated the entire neighborhood a county "crime hotspot" and directed multiple resources to the neighborhood. Nonetheless, in 2018, reported crime in Langley Park still exceeded that in the county (see Table 1). While property crimes per 1000 residents were similar between Langley Park and the county, violent crimes per 1,000 residents were over three times higher in Langley Park. Given its small geographic area, the gap in violent crime per 100 acres was even higher. This included gang activity, especially but not limited to MS-13, which inspired fear among residents (Miller & Morse, 2017).

While CASA's mission focuses on immigrant rights' advocacy, it had long been engaged in efforts to reduce crime and increase safety in Langley Park as part of its community development program. With CBCR funding for planning, CASA brought several organizations together under the Langley Park Crime Prevention Collaboration (CPC) starting in 2016. CPC members

Table 1. Crime by type per person and acre in Langley Park compared to Prince George County, 2018.

Crimes by Type per Person and Acre, 2018

Type	Prince George's County*			Langley Park CDP		
	Total	Crimes per 1,000 Persons	Crimes per 100 Acres	Total	Crimes per 1,000 Persons	Crimes per 100 Acres
Property Crimes	13,768	15.5	4.5	294	15.1	46.4
Violent Crimes	2,003	2.4	0.6	151	7.7	23.8
Total	15,771	18.2	5.1	445	22.8	70.2
Population	8,89,807	-	-	19,520	-	-
Acreage	3,08,921	-	-	634	-	-
Population Density per Acre	2.88	-	-	19,717	-	-

* Excludes Langley Park. Data source: Prince George's Police Department (2021) "Crime Incidents February 2017 to Present." Accessed at https://data.princegeorgescountymd.gov/Public-Safety/Crime-Incidents-February-2017-to-Present/wb4e-w4nf

included local politicians, university researchers, apartment managers, tenants, parents, faith-based leaders, representatives from other community-based organizations and county police.

CPC members, including university researchers, met monthly to identify public safety priorities and initiatives. Researchers also held focus groups with youth and police, conducted a community survey on residents' perceptions on public safety, analyzed neighborhood crime data, and convened a community town hall. Given feedback from these investigations, CPC members drew up an implementation plans focused largely on five neighborhood "crime hotspots". As a result of this robust planning, DOJ funded CPC's implementation plans in 2018. The final implementation plans identified four key problems: language and cultural differences between police and residents; a lack of trust between police and residents; unemployment and poverty that contribute to crime; and crime hotspots that undermine public safety. It proposed five key strategy areas to address these problems: (1) improve community-police relations; (2) increase neighborhood social cohesion; (3) alcohol-related crimes responses; (4) youth gang prevention and intervention; and (5) elimination of crime hotspots. Each strategy included multiple activities, success measures, and milestones.

Planned activities for the two-year implementation phase (2018–2020) to increase community-police relations included cultural competency and language training for officers, monthly "Coffee with an Officer" (*Club de Café*) community meetings, and a youth-police soccer league. The other strategies all focused on community capacity-building and neighborhood improvement. Planned activities included a community resource access campaign, an alcohol awareness program, a gang prevention program, community walks, and infrastructure upgrades.

Original figure can be viewed in the journal article. Copyright permission could not be obtained for this figure.

In the program's last year, some programs were changed or ended due to COVID-19. With poor housing conditions, high poverty rates, and many essential workers, Langley Park had some of the highest infection rates in the county and state (Green, 2020a). In March 2020, the *Club de Café*, community walks, and Spanish language classes were suspended. The gang prevention, alcoholism awareness, and youth soccer league programs transitioned to online activities, though the latter resumed in-person practices in summer 2020 CASA and CPC organizations also transitioned many of its resources to address immediate COVID relief, including a CASA-led Solidarity Fund to provide direct cash and food assistance to residents.

During the implementation phase, researchers attended monthly CPC meetings with residents and other stakeholders. They evaluated outcome data on each program, including participant surveys administered by CPC partners, and program materials and notes. For others, including language training for officers and the youth soccer league, researchers designed and administered surveys and focus groups. Each program was evaluated according to the objectives originally laid out in the approved grant, which varied for each program, but generally related to the number of participants or those reached, and some measure of impact, often assessed by pre- and post-surveys. After reviewing the data, researchers conducted six interviews with CPC partners to answer outstanding questions about program administration and implementation.[2] They also analyzed data from two CASA-led annual community surveys about overall project impacts. Finally, researchers tracked neighborhood crime data, integrating it with qualitative information drawn from community walks, and reported on public safety trends in Langley Park and its five hotspots to the CPC.

Community policing or investing in neighborhoods?

Given the implementation project's short timeframe, complications with COVID-19, data availability, and in some cases low participation rates, the success of individual programs was sometimes difficult to assess. Crime data and residents' changing perceptions of crime were particularly difficult areas in which to draw conclusive results.

During the CBCR implementation period, neither crime data nor residents' sense of safety markedly declined. Consistent with national trends, crime trended downwards or was flat for property and violent crime (see Figure 1). Before and after the start of the COVID-19 pandemic, the downward trend sharpened (Green, 2020a). According to the Division Police Commander, however, this was perhaps due in part to a reduced police presence and longer response times during the pandemic (Green, 2020b). Interestingly, a fifth of 2019 community survey respondents felt that crime had gotten worse in the past year; and in 2020, 43% of respondents felt the same. During the same period, the percentage of respondents who felt safe walking alone during the day increased only slightly, from 57% to 60%, while the percentage of those who felt unsafe walking alone at night increased from 86% to 98%. With low

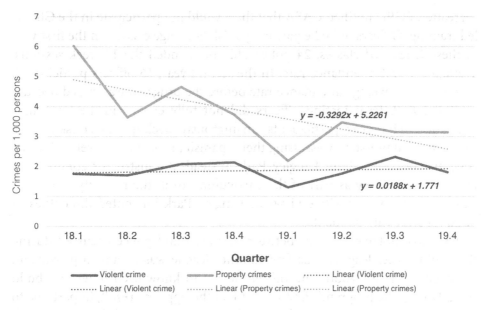

Figure 1. Crimes by type in Langley Park, 2018–2019.

survey participation rates, the findings were suggestive rather than conclusive, but still pointed to mixed reviews about residents' perceptions of crime and sense of safety.[3]

When comparing across multiple programs, however, the research showed differences in the success of programs designed to build community-police trust and those that invested in the neighborhood. The former often struggled with a lack of resident participation, police cooperation, and overall impacts. In contrast, investments in neighborhood infrastructure, resident education, resource access, and capacity- and community-building had more positive and potentially long-lasting results, including improved neighborhood quality and resident engagement in crime reduction strategies.

Building bonds between community and police

Several CBCR programs had the stated goal of building trust between residents and the Prince George's County police. Among all the project goals, this was the most challenging, in large part because of a lack of police participation and cooperation, longstanding fractured community-police relations, and ongoing incidents of police violence.

Planned CBCR programs for bridging police-community relations included cultural competency and language classes for officers. The former never took place. Before CBCR implementation PGPD and University of Maryland researchers unaffiliated with this project had a highly publicized debate about a cultural competency training that utilized virtual reality. Shortly thereafter, PGPD notified CASA that they would not participate in the CBCR-led training. Officers did take part in Spanish language classes. In the first year of these CASA-led classes, 24 police officers attended the 12-week sessions, averaging a 47% attendance rate. In the second year, 16 officers participated, with the same average attendance rate before the program was ended because of COVID-19. Participating officers did not fully engage in the program's evaluation. First-year participants unanimously declined to consent to a researcher-led pre-survey assessing their Spanish proficiency as well as knowledge and opinions about Langley Park. Instead, the instructor conducted a more limited survey as part of the curriculum. In it, the majority of officers expressed relatively positive views of Langley Park but noted difficulties in building trust with residents.

The most notable tensions between residents and police occurred during the youth soccer league. This free summer league was meant to provide an informal venue for youth and officers to get to know each other and build trust. During the program's first year, it had the opposite result, in part due to the program's structure and a lack of clear expectations. While a few officers attended practices, they were unclear about their expected roles and rarely played with youth. Youth characterized their interactions with police as patronizing, intrusive, and sometimes hostile. "Why do we need to have security?" asked one young boy. "We felt unsafe because they were just watching," noted another.[4] After discussions with coaches and police, CASA changed the structure of the program to assign police a clearer but less central role the following year and set explicit expectations for youth and officers. Police attended half of the practices, largely to share safety information with youth during structured water breaks, which did not allow time for them to engage informally. The changes lessened tensions between youth and police but did little to build trust or change residents' already negative perceptions of police. Instead, youth and parents characterized the program's successes as engaging youth in activities and allowing them to use a central neighborhood space (a designated local crime hotspot) often occupied by older youth. In all, 50 youth participated, exceeding the 25 to 35 for which CASA had planned.

Additionally, the Club de Café was designed with the goals of increasing trust between police officers and residents. However, like the youth soccer league, according to community participants and CASA leadership, the police largely used the monthly events to provide information to rather than interact with residents. Similarly, CASA staff also noted that the roles between officers and residents were unclear. A resident who helped to organize the events and recruit participants said they did little to change the distrust residents had of police. "They would still leave a bit worried about the police, and not completely satisfied with everything happening – the crime, and all the questions [the police] ask," she noted of residents. Toward the program's end, few residents showed up and those that did were often the same people.

Police-involved incidents that occurred during the CBCR implementation period further strained community-police relations. One particularly charged incident occurred early in 2020. The confrontation, which was caught on tape and widely shared across social media, involved a resident that appeared to be pushed down by an off-duty PGPD officer at a Langley Park shopping center. The officer, who was already involved in another internal affairs investigation, failed to help the resident who appeared unconscious (Morse, 2020). The incident fueled frustration in Langley Park, particularly as PGPD suspended, but did not charge the officer, after little communication with residents. Tensions were reignited months later when PGPD released a video showing an officer violently kicking a suspect at a Langley Park gas station (Davies & Weil, 2020). The video was released two months after the incident and multiple community requests. Its release corresponded with national uprisings around police violence, including many protests in Prince George's County. After PGPD communicated with CASA about the incidents, CASA staff shared information with residents, who were increasingly distrustful of information shared directly by police.

In the program's final months, police participation in CPC meetings waned and officers did not respond to repeated researcher invitations to participate in planned focus groups. According to community survey measures, community-police trust changed little, but improved slightly within a one-year period. In the implementation grant's first year, more than half (56%) of respondents felt uncomfortable reporting crime, in part because of fears of being treated unfairly by police, compared to 45% a year later. During the same period, the percentage who agreed that police did a good job addressing neighborhood problems went from 46% to 59%. Still, low survey participation rates make these apparent improvements difficult to assess in light of the negative experiences and opinions expressed by residents during the implementation phase.

Resourcing and educating the community

CASA designed multiple programs to improve residents' access to and education about community resources, including those associated with alcohol prevention and crime and safety. The programs were related to the goal of addressing the underlying factors that contribute to crime, such as residents' lack of access to ~~support systems related to~~ employment and mental health services.

The CPC created a community resource guide based on the needs of residents expressed in focus groups and surveys. CASA printed over 1,000 copies and their organizers distributed them door-to-door before COVID hit. This guide and outreach connected residents to educational, financial, health, social services, employment, workforce development, and language resources in addition to those about public safety, reflecting CASA's holistic community development approach.

The alcohol awareness program complemented the resource access campaign and built on CASA's nationally recognized health promoter (*promotora*) program. This program trains residents on health and risk-prevention strategies who then educate their neighbors, friends, and families. CASA health promoters visited shopping centers, liquor stores, and other gathering places to distribute fliers and speak to residents about the dangers of alcoholism, warning signs, and resources. They established a Facebook page to support and connect with residents. The program exceeded its goal of reaching 1,000 people by contacting over 1,500 people through social media, one-on-one conversations, and referrals. CASA also used community testimony and crime reports from CPC research partners to organize a successful campaign preventing the reissuance of a liquor license at a site of historic alcohol abuse and related crimes located in a locally designated crime hotspot.

As the pandemic took hold, DOJ permitted CASA to divert some CBCR funding for COVID relief. CASA staff provided masks, food, and rent relief to affected residents. Health promoters conducted public health outreach on social media, and followed up with residents to provide direct relief, including transportation to testing sites. These efforts underscored the position of the CPC that improving safety in Langley Park could not be achieved through a primary emphasis on policing. It also had to help address the basic needs of residents that, when not met, contribute to crime.

Improving neighborhood infrastructure

Working with the Neighborhood Design Center (NDC), a CPC partner, residents planned a variety of improvements to neighborhood spaces. They suggested widened sidewalks at a popular school bus stop; traffic-calming measures on dangerous roadways; areas for improved lighting; murals in common gathering spaces; and traffic box wraps that could turn everyday infrastructure into opportunities for community celebration.

Few of the projects were completed during the CBCR grant period, in part because of the time needed for coordination and implementation as well as DOJ funding restrictions. However, CASA leveraged the CPC to obtain additional county funding and commitments worth approximately $2 million. By late 2020, CASA and NDC had begun a tree planting program on private and public property; installing shrubs and fence pillars along popular pedestrian corridors; and planning for a community garden. They started a graffiti removal program and installed several vandalism-resistant art wraps on traffic and utility boxes (Figure 2). CASA hired and worked with local artists and

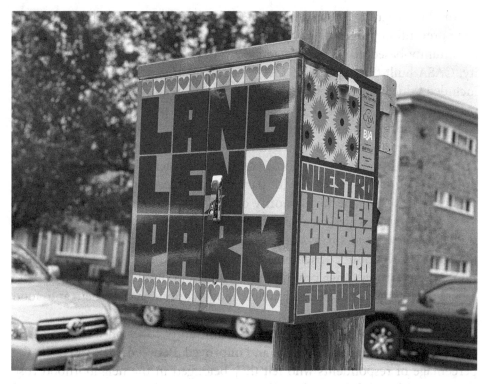

Figure 2. Langley Park traffic box art wrap. Hyattsville Community Development Corporation.

residents to install artwork at school bus stops, other high-traffic areas, and on storm drains. These projects continued beyond the formal grant period, a welcome sign of sustainability.

Building community capacity and cohesion

An important tenet of DOJ's CBCR grant program is that building social cohesion leads to a safer neighborhood. Planned activities leveraged and strengthened Langley Park's already strong sense of community and the capacities of its residents and organizations.

Eight community walks provided an effective venue for residents to learn about each other and the neighborhood. These walks brought residents, police, and other stakeholders through the locally designated crime hotspots to share information about and strategies to address crime and improve safety and infrastructure. They gave voice to residents' perceptions of safety and catalyzed action. While police attended several walks, they took a backseat to residents, listening to them about issues and solutions. Even so, the police presence dissuaded resident involvement. While some residents participated in the walks, according to its organizers, some others were "scared because neighbors would see them with the police."

Another program that built on the neighborhood's existing capacity was the gang prevention program, led by the Latin American Youth Center (LAYC), a community-based nonprofit. To address residents' concern about gang activity, CASA built the capacity of LAYC's existing after school program, which included education on college preparation, job readiness, health, and gang prevention. LAYC used CBCR funds to hire a new part-time staff member to support the program as an academic advisor. In the second year, funds were used to transition the position to a full-time program manager and help LAYC hire a workforce manager to boost youth employment. The gang prevention program had positive results, with participants exceeding the expected numbers in both years. The vast majority of participants demonstrated increased knowledge of strategies to avoid gang involvement and conflict resolution skills in standardized surveys taken upon their entry into and completion of the gang prevention curriculum. Equally importantly, the funding built LAYC's capacity in other program areas and supported their direct COVID relief, including outreach to families about computer, internet, and food assistance.

According to the community survey, community cohesion was high at the start of the implementation period and improved. Between 2019 and 2020, the percentage of respondents who felt they belonged in the neighborhood rose (71% to 85%) as did those who talked with their neighbors (65% to 86%) and had pride in the neighborhood (44% to 59%).

Conclusion: improving community safety by investing in neighborhoods

The CBCR planning and implementation grant offered an opportunity to improve community safety in Langley Park. Evaluation of the CPC's two-year implementation programs showed that neither neighborhood crime data nor sense of safety changed much. While there was inconclusive evidence as to whether the program met its primary goals of reducing crime and increasing police-community trust, programs that invested in building the capacity of this declining inner-ring suburb experienced more success. The latter generally met their stated program goals, and tended to have the most robust engagement. Some also remain ongoing after the grant period, including the youth soccer league (with no police involvement), LAYC gang prevention program, health promotion activities, and placemaking initiatives. In contrast, efforts focused on building trust with police often did not fully meet their goals and ended after CBCR funding stopped.

CASA's role was central to achieving the program's successes. As a high-capacity, community-based, advocacy organization, its staff leveraged their strong ties within and outside the neighborhood. Throughout the program, CASA staff's strong community ties helped to keep residents at the table and at the forefront of discussions about program planning. They transformed a grant focused on community policing to one that invested heavily in community development and built the capacity of residents and nonprofits, improved neighborhood conditions, and responded to residents' critical needs during the pandemic. They also faced similar challenges as residents in working with police. When tensions arose between residents and police, CASA acted as a mediator. Their work on immigrant rights nationally and locally sometimes put them at odds with police, particularly in the midst of national uprisings and anti-immigrant crackdowns.

Given the challenges of community policing efforts in Latinx immigrant neighborhoods, this study shows how funds currently used for policing Latinx neighborhoods might be better spent investing in building capacity and connections among community-based organizations and residents as well as leveraging their expertise for sustained community change. Like other studies, it confirms that investments in community-led, place-based initiatives help to reduce neighborhood crime and increase safety. But it adds to the limited strategies focused on inner-ring suburbs and Latinx immigrant communities, highlighting the need to invest in their aging infrastructure, educate and improve access residents' to existing resources, and build and leverage the capacity of existing residents and organizations. It also highlights the critical role of community-based organizations in helping residents imagine and execute programs that improve community safety without relying solely or even primarily on police.

Notes

1. All demographic statistics are from the U.S. Census Bureau, 2014–2018 American Community Survey Five-Year Estimates.
2. This research was conducted with the approval of the Institutional Review Board of University of Maryland, College Park, No. 1,447,513–1. Unless otherwise noted, all quotes come from interviews conducted by CPC researchers, October 2020. The purpose of interviews was largely to answer outstanding questions that researchers had about individual programs and their implementation after evaluating the data on each program. Interviews were conducted with the CPC Coordinator, the Spanish language instructor, a PGPD officer, two NDC staff members, and the youth soccer coach.
3. The community survey was written by researchers at the University of Maryland and administered by CASA staff in August to September 2019 and September to October 2020 at CBCR and other community events. The survey was available in both English and Spanish, and available online and in-person. Almost all participants completed the survey in-person and in Spanish. The 2020 survey was combined with a needs analysis of COVID-19-related resources. Outreach was hampered by the pandemic. Due to the low turnout rates, researchers did not conduct tests of statistical significance.
4. Quotes from youth focus groups conducted by CPC researchers, July 2019.

Acknowledgments

The authors wish to thank all the CPC members who diligently contributed to this effort, particularly those from CASA, including Alonzo Washington, Donta Council, Sara Rockefeller, and Julio Murillo. We also appreciate the guidance and support of the Local Initiatives Support Corporation, particularly Matt Perkins.

Disclosure statement

No potential conflict of interest was reported by the author(s).

Funding

This project was supported by Grant No. 2017-AJ-BX-0002 awarded by the Bureau of Justice Assistance. Points of view or opinions in this document are those of the author and do not necessarily represent the official position or policies of the U.S. Department of Justice.

References

Alexander, M. (2011). *The new jim crow: Mass incarceration in the age of colorblindness*. New Press.

Chaney, C., & Robertson, R. V. (2013). Racism and police brutality in America. *Journal of African American Studies*, 17(4), 480–505. https://doi.org/10.1007/s12111-013-9246-5

Davies, E., & Weil, M. (2020, June 3). Three Prince George's County officers suspended after suspect kicked, police say. . https://www.washingtonpost.com/local/public-safety/three-prince-georges-county-officers-suspended-after-suspect-kicked-police-say/2020/06/03/dca55e0e-a54d-11ea-bb20-ebf0921f3bbd_story.html.

Garcia-Hallett, J., Like, T., Torres, T., & Irazábal, C. (2020). Latinxs in the Kansas City metro area: Policing and criminalization in ethnic enclaves. *Journal of Planning Education and Research*, 40(2), 151–168. https://doi.org/10.1177/0739456X19882749

Gilmore, R. W. (2007). *Golden gulag: Prisons, surplus, crisis, and opposition in globalizing California*. University of California Press.

Green, R. (2020a). *COVID-19 and reported crime in Langley Park: A briefing paper for the community-based crime prevention program of CASA*. Report to Langley Park Crime Prevention Collaborative. Howard University.

Green, R. (2020b). *Crime levels, trends, and recommendations for the Langley Park target area and five hotspots*. Report to Langley Park Crime Prevention Collaborative. Howard University.

Hipple, N., & Saunders, J. (2020). *Evaluation of the innovation in community-based crime reduction (CBCR) program* (Report No. 254623). Indiana University. https://www.ncjrs.gov/pdffiles1/nij/grants/254623.pdf.

Lane, M., & Henry, K. (2004). Beyond symptoms: Crime prevention and community development. *Australian Journal of Social Issues*, 39(2), 201–213. https://doi.org/10.1002/j.1839-4655.2004.tb01172.x

Lung-Amam, W., Pendall, R., & Knaap, E. (2019). Mi casa no es su casa: Transit-induced gentrification and the fight for equitable development in an inner-ring, immigrant suburb. *Journal of Planning Education and Research*, 39(4), 442–455. https://doi.org/10.1177/0739456X19878248

Martinez, R. (2002). *Latino homicide: Immigration, violence, and community*. Routledge.

Miller, M., & Morse, D. (2017). 'People here live in fear': MS-13 menaces a community seven miles from the White House. The Washington Post. https://www.washingtonpost.com/local/people-here-live-in-fear-ms-13-menaces-a-community-seven-miles-from-the-white-house/2017/12/20/6cebf318-d956-11e7-b859-fb0995360725_story.html.

Morse, D. (2020, April 15). Prince George's police officer suspended after confrontation outside liquor store. https://www.washingtonpost.com/local/public-safety/prince-georges-police-officer-suspended-after-confrontation-outside-liquor-store/2020/04/15/aafb375e-7f4e-11ea-9040-68981f488eed_story.html.

Naughton, J. (1991, August 19) Hispanics carve niche in P.G. *The Washington Post*. https://www.washingtonpost.com/archive/politics/1991/08/19/hispanics-carve-niche-in-pg/98a4c030-736a-4e97-bf31-a46c6d5837e8/.

Roth, B. J., & Grace, B. (2018). Structural barriers to inclusion in a Latino immigrant new destination: Exploring the adaptive strategies of social service organizations in South Carolina. *Journal of International Migration and Integration*, 19(4), 1075–1093. https://doi.org/10.1007/s12134-018-0587-8

Saint-Fort, P., Yasso, N., & Shah, S. (2012). Engaging police in immigrant communities: Promising practices from the fiel. Vera Institute for Justice. https://www.vera.org/downloads/Publications/engaging-police-in-immigrant-communities-promising-practices-from-the-field/legacy_downloads/engaging-police-in-immigrant-communities.pdf

Sampson, R. J., & Loeffler, C. (2010). Punishment's place: The local concentration of mass incarceration. *Daedalus*, 139(3), 20–31. https://doi.org/10.1162/DAED_a_00020

Simpson, S. A., Steil, J., & Mehta, A. (2020). Planning beyond mass incarceration. *Journal of Planning Education and Research*, 40(2), 130–138. https://doi.org/10.1177/0739456X20915505

Skogan, W. G. (2006). The promise of community policing. In D. L. Weisburd & A. A. Braga (Eds.), *Police innovation: Contrasting perspectives* (pp. 27–44). Cambridge University.

Stein, R. E., & Griffith, C. (2015). Resident and police perceptions of the neighborhood: Implications for community policing. *Criminal Justice Police Review*, 28(2), 130–138. https://doi.org/10.1177/0887403415570630

Xie, M., & Baumer, E. P. (2019). Neighborhood immigrant concentration and violent crime reporting to the police: A multilevel analysis of data from the national crime victimization survey. *Criminology*, 57(2), 237–267. https://doi.org/10.1111/1745-9125.12204

Bursting bubbles: outcomes of an intergroup contact intervention within the context of a community based violence intervention program

Christopher St. Vil and Kwasi Boaitey

ABSTRACT

Intergroup contact theory has received much quantitative support. However few efforts have attempted to apply qualitative methodologies to understand the perceptions of individuals who experience these contacts. we conducted 19 interviews to explore the perceptions of stakeholders of a community-based fitness program whose goal was to increase intergroup contact among its stakeholders. Participants reflected on the program reducing their social isolation, increasing opportunities for engagement outside one's own group, and expanded world views.

Background

Racism and prejudice continue to be an enduring issue in U.S. society (Dominelli, 2018). Much of the prejudice between varying racial groups persists because of government-based sanctioning of housing segregation which kept American citizens from meaningful engagement across race (Imbroscio, 2020; Rothstein, 2017). Specifically, this segregation was targeted at keeping African Americans/Blacks from interacting with Whites and reinforced concentrations of Black poverty and White affluence (Howell, 2019; Johnson, 2008; Wilson, 1987). From a human service perspective, given the psychological impact of prejudice (Major & Vick, 2005), it is imperative that organizations actively integrate anti-racist practices both within their organizations (Ferguson, 2008; Nnawulezi et al., 2016) and throughout their provision of services (James, 1996; Santiago & Ivery, 2020). There are numerous ways organizations can engage in anti-racist work (Dominelli, 2018). One form of anti-racist work is increasing the level of intergroup contact with the goal of reducing prejudice and bias and increasing understanding (Allport, 1954), especially among Whites and minoritized populations in the United

States. A key mechanism on which intergroup contact theory is based is the assumption that if members of different and often segregated groups come together, intergroup relations will improve.

Intergroup contact theory

Allport's (1954) formulation of intergroup contact theory was a coalescence of research that took place during the 1930s and 40s exploring the impact of intergroup exposure on individuals' attitudes toward different ethnic groups (Loader, 2015). A summary of that body of research suggested contact with Black Americans produced more positive racial attitudes among White Americans under specific conditions (T. F. Pettigrew, 1998). Using this research as a framework, Allport formulated a hypothesis arguing that intergroup contact only reduces prejudice in situations that meet four optimal conditions: equal group status within the contact situation, common goals, intergroup cooperation, and the support of authorities, law, or customs (Allport, 1954; Christ & Kauff, 2019). A meta-analysis of this body of work offered several conclusions regarding conditions that reduced prejudice through intergroup contact (Pettigrew & Tropp, 2006). First, intergroup contact can contribute meaningfully to reductions in prejudice across a broad range of groups and contexts. Second, although empirical studies that incorporated Allport's optimal conditions into their models reported higher effect sizes, Allport's conditions were not essential for intergroup contact to achieve positive outcomes. Overall, the body of literature unequivocally supports the idea that interventions seeking to reduce racial prejudice through intergroup contact are, in fact, effective.

Research exploring intergroup contact since Allport's (1954) work has been pervasive, however, it has tended to be quantitative, with laboratory studies garnering the highest value (Loader, 2015). A meta-analysis yielded 526 quantitative papers resulting in 713 independent samples between 1940 and 2000 alone (Pettigrew & Tropp, 2006). However, this overreliance on quantitative methods has limited our understanding of how intergroup contacts manifest in the real world and how the actors in these contacts perceive the interactions themselves (Dixon et al., 2005; Loader, 2015). Although the number of studies exploring intergroup contact with qualitative methods remains small, the few that have been conducted have shed light in how intergroup contact operates in everyday settings (Loader, 2015). These studies have focused on a variety of cultural contexts such as Muslims (Blackwood et al., 2013), the Maori and Pakeha of New Zealand (Fozdar, 2011), university students (Halualani, 2008), Arab and Jewish children in bilingual schools in Israel (Hughes, 2007), South Africans on beaches (Dixon & Durrheim, 2003), Catholic and Protestant children in Northern Ireland (Loader, 2015), and employees with disabilities (Novak et al., 2011). This study seeks to build on this body of literature by presenting the results of a qualitative inquiry into the impact of an intergroup contact intervention within the context of a community-based gun violence program. The purpose of this study is to present the findings of qualitative inquiries among participants within the Inner-City Weightlifting program about their experiences with forming relationships with individuals of different racial and class backgrounds.

Program description

Inner City Weightlifting (ICW) is a nonprofit organization established in Boston, Massachusetts in 2010 (Malamut, 2013). The stated goal and purpose of ICW is to curb gun violence and ICW works toward this goal by extending opportunities for economic mobility and social inclusion to individuals who have engaged in gun violence and/or experienced incarceration. The organization helps these individuals achieve economic mobility by teaching them to become physical trainers, hence the moniker, ICW. Physical fitness is the main activity that facilitates the development of rapport between the organization and its students. When a potential student joins ICW, they matriculate through a four-stage process that includes pursuing their physical trainer certifications and forming relationships with their gym clients to create social capital.

ICW is a merging of two passions: fitness and social justice. While the track to becoming a physical trainer fulfills the fitness passion, the second passion of social justice is grounded in improving the plight of Black and Brown men from marginalized communities and eradicating racism, stigmatization, and prejudice through anti-racism work. This is manifested through the deliberate pairing of the students with their clients at Stage 3. To an observer, it appears that the intention of this match is for the benefit of the student. However, the real intention of the pairing according to the ICW staff is the expansion of the world view of the client and a reduction in their bias toward Black and Brown men specifically, and Black and Brown communities in general.

Participants and procedures

Seeking IRB approval and solidifying the planning for the study in terms of the design and instrumentation transpired during the Spring and Summer of 2018. Data collection for this study occurred across two groups of informants: students and their clients. ICW students were recruited remotely. Flyers targeting the students were posted around the ICW gym for students to be aware of the opportunity to engage in a semi-structured interview about their experience with the program. Those students who had e-mail addresses also received the flyer via e-mail. Additionally, word got around the gym that a researcher was coming to interview students who were willing to talk about

Table 1. # of interview participants by role and interview length.

Role	# of participants	Hours of Audio
Students	10	5 h 12 m (312 minutes)
Gym Clients	9	2 h 33 m (153 minutes)
Total	19	
Hours of audio		7 h 45 m

their experience with ICW. If the ICW staff did not identify a prospective individual respondent as a student, they would have been excluded from the potential pool of students eligible to be interviewed. The recruitment solicitation of gym clients to participate in focus group discussions took place through e-mail. All gym clients had a functional e-mail account that eliminated the need for phone calls and alternative forms of recruitment. A separate e-mail solicitation was created for the gym clients which an ICW staff member distributed through the client listserv. Follow-up correspondence regarding the study was directed to me or a research assistant via e-mail. Focus groups were conducted in a closed office at the Harvard Square site. Semi-structured interviews occurred in an available room/office at either the Harvard or Dorchester program sites.

The focus group discussion guide was comprised of 6–8 questions that focused on client experiences with their trainers and how their views/perspectives of Black and Hispanic men from marginalized neighborhoods may have changed as a result of their experience with ICW. The semi-structured interview guide for the trainers included 12 questions that focused on their history, how they came to join ICW, and their mentorship experiences. We proceeded to plan logistically for scheduling the in-person semi-structured interviews and focus groups. Students were the only interview participants who received a stipend for their time.

In total, the study collected data from 19 individuals for a total of 7 hours and 45 minutes of audio recorded content. Table 1 reveals that there were 10 student semi-structured interviews, and 2 focus groups that consisted of 9 clients. The age range for the nine gym clients shown in Table 2 was between 29 and 80 with a mean age of 47. Most of the gym clients who participated in the focus group were female. All but two of the gym clients reported graduate

Table 2. Select demographics of gym clients.

Name	Age	Gender	Occupation	Education
Gym Client A	80	F	Investment Analyst (R)	MBA
Gym Client B	54	M	Product Manager in Hi – Tech field	Bachelors
Gym Client C	58	F	Gerentologist	Masters
Gym Client D	29	F	Social Worker	Masters
Gym Client E	51	F	Life Coach	JD
Gym Client F	29	F	Systems Engineer	Bachelors
Gym Client G	61	F	Lawyer	JD
Gym Client H	31	M	Software Engineer	Doctorate
Gym Client I	31	F	Director Bio-tech company	Masters

BEYOND LIP SERVICE

Table 3. Select demographics of the student group (n = 10).

Name	Age	Race
Student 1	21	AA
Student 2	26	AA
Student 3	25	AA
Student 4	26	AA
Student 5	23	His
Student 6	33	AA
Student 7	30	His
Student 8	31	His
Student 9	34	His
Student 10	31	AA

level degrees and they held a variety of occupations. Data on the students are presented in Table 3. Student participants in the study were 28 years old on, average, and six self-identified as African American/Black and 4 self-identified as Hispanic.

Analysis

The data for this study involved semi-structured interviews with the students and focus groups with the gym clients with whom the students were matched. After transcription, all interviews were read independently and openly coded, consistent with a grounded theory approach (Glaser & Strauss, 1999). After all transcripts were read and coded independently, the authors met to reconciliate the free codes and arrive at agreement on a coding scheme. A second read through of all transcripts was conducted using the agreed upon coding scheme. The research team regrouped to discuss and reconcile the themes that emerged repeatedly from the coding scheme. After team deliberations, three themes emerged from these interviews associated with the research questions of this paper: (1) community building; (2) enhancement of social networks; and (3) beyond training/toward understanding. In the discussion of the generated themes, pseudonyms are used instead of actual names.

Results

Community building

ICW seeks institutional change through (1) providing opportunities to young men from communities plagued by gun violence with case management and career opportunities, and (2) challenging racial and class stereotypes through the purposeful matching of students with physical fitness clients from the opposite socioeconomic background with the goal of expanding the network of both clients and students. Inherent in the mission is the idea of community building between individuals who otherwise would not have had the opportunity to meet each other. Mario, who has been a trainer at ICW for just under ten years, stated when they went to events: "I realized that – I mean he's [ICW staff] putting us in a position where we're meeting people we would never meet otherwise." Mario went on to say:

> How I explain it straight up is just I met White people that I never even would meet before. Rich White people. You know what I'm saying? That's it. You know what I mean? I felt like—it wasn't just White people. It was a bunch of people, you know, but it was the majority of White people. You know what I'm saying? I'm like, "Damn, this is like I would never meet these people." I felt like this could be connections to other things. You know what I mean? I felt like I could network properly if I went this avenue, so I stuck with it. You know what I mean?

Here, Mario is expressing his perceived recognition of the ICW staff trying to improve his social network and social capital by putting him in a position to develop relationships with individuals he never thought he would have an opportunity to do so otherwise. Another trainer Donald expressed a similar sentiment:

> Then I was just like, 'Al'ight, but what am I doin' while I'm here? Am I just gonna work out?' That's when we started meetin' these people from these affluent backgrounds . . . Like I said, that bridging them back out because relationships—that shit is big, yo. To me anyway, 'cause there are some influential people here and they rub shoulders with other influential people, and if you can just plant a seed over there that yo, we're not that bad. We al'ight over here. Some of us might need—the way this shit's designed, we might need a little help to come up out this shit because this was by design?

Here, Donald invokes the concept of "bridging." He understands the opportunity he has to develop relationships with individuals he views not only as affluent but as influential. Donald's comment also reflected his thoughts of not wanting to be viewed from the stigma of the "Black criminal stereotype" (Welch, 2007) which he views as so pervasive.

While the expressed need for an expansion of social capital and a social network is evident among the students, this same sentiment was also expressed among the clients, albeit, for different reasons. Carole expressed her feelings about segregation as a barrier to community building in this way:

> I feel like my ability or my opportunities to interact with people from different places, different backgrounds is getting more and more limited as the dynamic in this country changes, and we really don't interact a lot. I think that what—we were just talking about this with DC, right? DC with the changing of the neighborhood. Where you would have a neighborhood before that was multi-generational, and diverse, and multi-socioeconomical, we don't have that anymore. We have rich people; we have poor people. We have Black people; we have White people.

Carole described her ability to experience a diverse group of people as being constrained by the bifurcation of society into the haves and have nots. One Client, George, stated, "this is where I have exposure to people who are not in the bubble of life that I'm in," which also suggests a separation of sort.

A client named Shawn made this comment when asked the same question:

... one thing I've been struggling with in Boston is that it is so segregated ... It made me realize just how white Boston is, and I think the thing I've been missing is: Where is a community of people who are just coming from different experiences than myself?

Both the students and the clients experienced a sense of isolation and segregation in their daily lives that made it unlikely they would have the opportunity to interact and meet people of a races and class different from their own outside of the gym. ICW's facilitation of the gym space allows for these unlikely relationships to form and approximates a form of community building based on reliance, working together on concrete fitness tasks and creating human, family, and social capital that provides a base for a new type of community.

Enhancement of social networks

The social networks of both the students and the clients expanded because of their involvement with ICW. These relationships with their origin in the gym were also robust outside of the gym. One of the trainers, Hassan, describes his experience with receiving support while being incarcerated:

I end up goin' to prison for three years. But I was the first to train a real client. Her name was [Sabrina] ... She helped me down on my situation, too, when I was in jail for the whole three years, come and visit me, write me, send me money, all of that. You know what I mean?

Hassan and the client are still connected and it's been over ten years since they first met. Mario had a similar experience as Hassan with being supported throughout his incarceration. After Mario returned home from prison and started working again at ICW, he began forming relationships with his clients that expanded beyond the gym:

Some of them give me jobs. Like one dude, I was down and out, one of my clients, he said his mom needed help moving, and gave his mom my number, and the mom called me, and I helped her move. You know what I mean? It's just networking. It's very big. You need that [in] life. I really don't have nobody to help me like that.

While the students expanded their network through building rapport with their clients, the clients expanded their network through the incorporation of the Black and Hispanic students into theirs. George expands on this below:

What I found is that when I started working with the gentleman here by the name of [Jeffrey], and we found a lot—I wasn't expecting to dive into it, but we found a lot of common ground areas such as being parents, relationships, outlook, sports, maybe music. I thought I had—really, then that benefit for me is not only am I getting better physically, but also from my relationship with people, people of color.

George saw value in including a formerly incarcerated Hispanic male into his network and perceived it as value added. Carole refers to an incident where she felt supported by a trainer in her network:

> I do know, I was in a grocery store once, Star, in Lower Mills. I was in line, and one of the guys from the gym was there. There was this Black woman who was in back of me. She was giving me shit over something. It was ridiculous. Like in a bad way. She was just being a jerk to me. He came over, and he gave me this big hug. Her mouth dropped. Like, you're friends with this guy from the hood? It just completely changed the dynamics. That was a great moment for me, because—and I think it was a great moment for him, because I felt like oh my god, this is my friend. He felt like I'm her friend, I'm gonna stick up for her.

Here, Carole describes how her relationship with one of the ICW trainers afforded her an amount of social and cultural capital that legitimized her and helped her defuse a tense situation in which the perpetrator adjusted their stance toward her because of that legitimization. The quotes offered by both the clients and students above suggest that the expansion of the network was beneficial to both parties. Additionally, the activities that undergirded the expansion of the networks did not take place in the gym. Two of the trainers described support from clients while incarcerated and one of the clients experienced the support of one of the trainers sporadically in a grocery store. This demonstrates that although the initiation of the relationship begins in the gym, the salience of the relationship reaches well beyond it.

Beyond training/toward understanding

ICW is attempting to play a role in eradicating racism by creating lasting bonds between

individuals who would not have done so under ordinary circumstances. This bond between students and clients is precisely what ICWs approach is suggesting leads to the critical shift in perspectives. Here, Donald gives his perspective on his changing views on class: "I don't think my perspective on race changed. My perspective on rich White people changed." Although it is not clear what Donald's views were about rich White people before ICW, it appears to have changed for the better.

Hassan also expresses his appreciation for his exposure to the world and for the program being instrumental in changing his life. He states, "what I say about that is because [Steven], he's in the citizen world and at the same time opened my eyes about changin' my life, you know what I mean, gettin' my GED, movin' on the right path." Hassan's use of the term "citizen world" refers to the mainstream formal economy which he distinguishes from the informal underground economy that he is well familiar with. His experiences with ICW helped change his perspective on life which led him to improve his education as well as his access to various forms of capital.

Another trainer, Jesus, who has been a trainer for ICW about 9 years spoke of his transition under one of the staff:

> I think he introduced me to a whole different world outside the streets. I remember being up on the top of the floor, just some tall buildings up in downtown. You lookin' out the windows, the views. It was stuff like that that opened my eyes. Then when he won an award for some shit ... he told me, he's like, "Yo, go get your passport." I'm like, "Motherfucker, how do I do that?" He helped me get my passport, we flew into Puerto Rico, and then after that we did a day in ... It just amazed me. I'm from a whole different world. I'm from the city projects, the shootings, the drugs, the crack heads around, the broken families ... When I seen that, that shit was like, "Wow, this is crazy, man.

From the client perspective, Laura, who describes herself as a middle-aged, White women from a well-educated family stated that her whole perspective of the criminal justice system changed because of her interaction with ICW.

> I have found my perception of how the justice system works, or doesn't work, has completely changed from what I thought it was, or what I learned it was growing up. I don't think it's a slam dunk anymore. I think there's always way more to the story. I actually happen to know somebody who had been arrested, and he's in this case, and they're not going to hear the case for a couple of years. Now I know, it's a terrible way to have to live your life, waiting. Being free, but not being free. Going out, waiting to try to carve out a life, and figuring out that it's just much more difficult, and then the attitude of some of the cops.

While Laura's view of the criminal justice system was impacted, another client Michelle explained how her experience with ICW has led her to begin to shift how she views Black men:

> I think, too, I look at people that I might've used to be afraid of, like on the bus or in the train, as human beings a little bit more. I think, as females, you're automatically pretty scared of all men *[laughter]* for a lot of reasons. It's just kind of ingrained in you but coming here and learning that they're not all out to get you, but particularly, big Black men aren't necessarily all out to get you, I think has been a pretty big perspective shift. I try to think more of, you know, what? They might look a little scary, but so does Angel sometimes. *[Laughter]* He is actually really gentle at heart, and just trying to be open to that, and that they're probably not the evil people that the world wants to make you think that they are.

Lastly, Roslyn shares the shift in her perspective because of attending ICW:

> I had a lot of things to overcome in a sense, or to confront all these past things that were not true, but I inherited. I had to, first of all, recognize I had them. Then, what was I gonna do about them? The other thing that I found is that I have viewed, in my actions towards Black people, I've changed. Because I'm no longer afraid of them. I see the good part of them. I've experienced the good part. Now, when go around or whatever someone holds the door a little bit for me, I am positive that I'm going to say thank you. I do anyhow, but especially if it's a Black person. Because I think, maybe I'm wrong, but I

think that Black people are not accustomed to expecting this type of courtesy or recognition from a lot of White people. I just figure I'm gonna be sure that I act courteously towards these people.

Discussion

Intergroup theory suggests that contact with minoritized individuals produces more positive racial attitudes among White Americans under certain conditions. In order to better understand how intergroup contexts manifest in the real world and how the individuals involved in such contacts perceive the interactions themselves, qualitative interviews were conducted with program participants of a community-based violence intervention program. Overall, the findings suggest that the intergroup contact facilitated by ICW resulted in a shift in the worldview and attitudes of the clients. For example, some clients stated that they hold a more critical view of the criminal justice system after hearing about the experiences of some students and some have promised to reach out to more Black people now that they no longer see them as a threat. Additionally, the data suggest that the shift in attitudes of the clients also extended in some cases to individuals beyond the students themselves thus having a positive impact on how the clients viewed other minoritized individuals outside of the students at-large. Further, the shift in attitudes of the students included shifts in views around race and class as well as behavior changes that included desistance of crime. These findings suggest that the anti-racist efforts of the organization were effective in helping shift the views and behaviors of both parties. In addition to perspective shifting, contact between the students and clients resulted in community building and social network enhancement. Within the context of these three themes all four of Allport's (1954) conditions are visible within ICWs approach.

First, the condition of "common goals" is manifested through the emphasis on the activity of fitness. As a result, the relationships between the students and clients revolve around the client's fitness goals for which the student is invested. Second, the condition of intergroup cooperation without competition is inherent through the student-client relationship in the gym and the effort of both parties to further the relationship outside the fitness context and push the boundaries around stereotypes. Both students and clients want each other to succeed. Third, because this relationship is initiated under the sanctioning of the ICW organization, the norms under which the trainer-client relationship develops is established and supported by the authority of the program staff which serve as a form of structural support and encouragement. Lastly, Allport argues that it is important for "equal group status" to precede reduction in prejudice. While it can be argued that the student and clients were not of equal status socio-economically or in regard to fitness knowledge, these are not the characteristics in which equality was achieved. Rather, it was achieved with the willingness of both parties to show up, be present and interact with each other with the goal of learning about each other. Both the clients and students are fully aware of the purpose of ICW which is to bring people together. Prejudice reduction requires an active, goal-oriented effort that leads to some sort of frequent sustained contact (T. F. Pettigrew, 1998). Thus, equality was achieved in their openness to each other and their willingness to be vulnerable to forming a relationship with someone that they otherwise would not have interacted with outside of the ICW context.

In a city characterized by social isolation and segregation, ICW goes beyond lip service by serving as a small oasis for individuals to interact and challenge biases and preconceived notions. ICWS approach address two of the 12 Grand Challenges of Social Work. It addresses smart decarceration through their reputation of working with students during and post- incarceration and it reduces extreme economic inequality by providing employment training, licensure and opportunities to a demographic that traditionally has a difficult time obtaining and sustaining employment.

Several lessons can be drawn from ICW for programs seeking to mirror these results. First, while the focus of ICW is on race relations, a program like this can be replicated for other issues that divide people, such as sexuality, politics, or religion. The main point is that there needs to be an activity that requires the actors to meet at some level of frequency; a sort of social arrangement that brings people together and reduces isolation. Second, organizations must be explicit in its marketing materials that it seeks to deliberately bring people together around an activity toward a goal or ideal. ICW makes clear on their website that it is not just a gym, but a place where people gain unique insight through personal connection thereby making the organization's goals clear to all participants. Third, the ICW staff engage in nudging (Hummel & Maedche, 2019) to methodically and strategically encourage both the clients and the students to explore interests outside of the gym and outside of fitness. Although the evidence around nudging is mixed, it is precisely this sort of encouragement that is thought to make the difference. Lastly, it has been suggested that all four of Allport's conditions are not essential for reducing prejudice and that these conditions are merely parts of a package that facilitate the effect of bias reduction (T.F. Pettigrew, 2008). Although all four conditions were present in this study, organizations need not wait for the condition to be present to implement their approach. These lessons can provide the basis for meaningful activities geared toward promoting cross race and cross class engagement.

This study compliments a larger body of qualitative work exploring the impact of intergroup contact theory and sheds some light on what actually goes on during the contact from the perspective of the actors themselves. In spite of this contribution, the study has its limitations. First, the findings from this study are derived from one program. The results and outcomes of this program cannot be extrapolated or hypothesized to operate similarly across other programs. Future qualitative research on the outcomes of intergroup contact theory should explore whether these themes emerge as salient in other contexts that may have opportunities to bring individuals of different racial backgrounds together such as afterschool programs and undergraduate college programs. Additionally, the self-selection of both the students and the clients for the interviews may have influenced the results. All clients do not engage in activities outside the gym with the students and all students do not get along perfectly with all clients, suggesting that self-selection may have introduced some bias by relying on program participants who possessed an overly positive outlook on the program. Future research would benefit from including the voices of those program participants who no longer frequent the gym as well as those who choose not to volunteer for such studies. A lack of these voices prevents an understanding of reasons for nonparticipation or reluctance to participate among clients.

In spite of these limitations, this study contributes to a growing body of qualitative work that seeks to explore the experiences of individuals engaged in relationships and programs with the goal of bias reduction. During this charged period in U.S. history fueled by divisive issues such as voting rights, critical race theory, and police use of force, it is incumbent among social service organizations that they begin to explore ways to incorporate anti-racist messaging and strategies into their approaches. With such a range of issues driving race to the forefront of political and social discourse, ICW provides one example of an initiative bursting the bubble of racism that currently grips our society.

Disclosure statement

No potential conflict of interest was reported by the author(s).

References

Allport, G. (1954). *The nature of prejudice*. Addison-Wesley.
Blackwood, L., Hopkins, N., & Reicher, S. (2013). "I know who I am, but who do they think I am?" Muslim perspectives on encounters with airport authorities. *Ethnic and Racial Studies*, 36(6), 1090–1108. https://doi.org/10.1080/01419870.2011.645845
Christ, O., & Kauff, M. (2019). Intergroup contact theory. In K. Sassenberg & M. L. W. Vliek (Eds.), *Social psychology in action: Evidence-based interventions from theory to practice* (pp. 145–161). Springer.
Dixon, J., Durrheim, K., & Tredoux, C. (2005). Beyond the optimal contact strategy: A reality check for the contact hypothesis. *American Psychologist*, 60(7), 697–711. https://doi.org/10.1037/0003-066X.60.7.697

Dixon, J., & Durrheim, K. (2003). Contact and the ecology of racial division: Some varieties of informal segregation. *British Journal of Social Psychology*, 42(1), 1–23. https://doi.org/10.1348/014466603763276090

Dominelli, L. (2018). *Anti-racist social work*. Palgrave.

Ferguson, S. A. (2008). Towards an anti-racist social service organization. *Journal of Multicultural Social Work*, 4(1), 35–48. https://doi.org/10.1300/J285v04n01_03

Fozdar, F. (2011). "I've never looked at someone and thought what colour they are": Contact theory and interracial friendship in New Zealand. *Journal of Intercultural Studies*, 32(4), 383–405. https://doi.org/10.1080/07256868.2011.584616

Glaser, B. G., & Strauss, A. L. (1999). *The discovery of grounded theory: Strategies for qualitative research*. Routledge.

Halualani, R. T. (2008). How do multicultural university students define and make sense of intercultural contact? A qualitative study. *International Journal of Intercultural Relations*, 32 (1), 1–16. https://doi.org/10.1016/J.IJINTREL.2007.10.006

Howell, J. (2019). The truly advantaged: Examining the effect of privileged places on educational attainment. *The Sociological Quarterly*, 60(3), 420–438. https://doi.org/10.1080/00380253.2019.1580546

Hughes, J. (2007). Mediating and moderating effects of inter-group contact: Case studies from bilingual/bi-national schools in Israel. *Journal of Ethnic and Migration Studies*, 3(3), 419–437. https://doi.org/10.1080/13691830701234533

Hummel, D. & Maedche, A. (2019). How effective is nudging? A quantitative review on the effect sizes and limits of emprical nudging. *Journal of Behavioral and Experimental Economics*, 80, 47–58.

Imbroscio, D. (2020). Race matters (even more than you already think): Racism, housing, and the limits of the Color of Law. *Journal of Race Ethnicity and the City*, 2(1), 29–53. https://doi.org/10.1080/26884674.2020.1825023

James, C. E. (1996). *Perspectives on racism and the human services sector: A case for change*. University of Toronto Press.

Johnson, O. (2008). Who benefits from concentrated affluence? A synthesis of neighborhood effects considering race, gender, and education outcomes. *Journal of Public Management and Social Policy*, 14(2), 85–112.

Loader, R. (2015). *Shared education in Northern Ireland: A qualitative study of intergroup contact* [Doctoral dissertation]. Queen's University Belfast. https://pure.qub.ac.uk/en/studentTheses/shared-education-in-northern-ireland-a-qualitative-study-of-inter

Major, B., & Vick, S. B. (2005). The psychological impact of prejudice. In J. F. Dovidio, P. Glick, & L. A. Rudman (Eds.), *On the nature of prejudice: Fifty years after Allport* (pp. 139–154). Blackwell.

Malamut, M. (2013, August 8). From the streets to the gym. *Boston Magazine*. https://www.bostonmagazine.com/health/2013/08/19/innercity-weightlifting-boston/

Nnawulezi, N., Ryan, A. M., & O'Connor, R. C. (2016). Reducing prejudice within community-based organizations. *Journal of Community Practice*, 24(2), 182–204. https://doi.org/10.1080/10705422.2016.115741

Novak, J., Feyes, K. J., & Christensen, K. A. (2011). Application of intergroup contact theory to the integrated workplace: Setting the stage for inclusion. *Journal of Vocational Rehabilitation*, 35(3), 211–226. https://doi.org/10.3233/JVR-2011-0573

Pettigrew, T. F., & Tropp, L. R. (2006). A meta-analytic test of intergroup theory. *Journal of Personality and Social Psychology*, 90(5), 751–783. https://doi.org/10.1037/0022-3514.90.5.751

Pettigrew, T. F. (1998). Intergroup contact theory. *Annual Review of Psychology*, 49(1), 65–85. https://doi.org/10.1146/annurev.psych.49.1.65

Pettigrew, T. F. (2008). Future directions for intergroup contact theory and research. *International Journal of Intercultural Relations*, 32(3), 187–199. https://doi.org/10.1016/j.ijintrel.2007.12.002

Rothstein, R. (2017). *The color of law: A forgotten history of how our government segregated America.* Liveright Publishing.

Santiago, A. M., & Ivery, J. (2020). Removing the knees from their necks: Mobilizing community practice and social action for racial justice. *Journal of Community Practice*, 28(3), 195–207. https://doi.org/10.1080/10705422.2020.1823672

Welch, K. (2007). Black criminal stereotypes and racial profiling. *Journal of Contemporary Criminal Justice*, 23(3), 276–288. https://doi.org/10.1177/1043986207306870

Wilson, W. J. (1987). *The truly disadvantaged: The inner city, the underclass, and public policy.* University of Chicago Press.

Can preference policies advance racial justice?

Amie Thurber (iD), Lisa K. Bates (iD), and Susan Halverson

ABSTRACT

Mitigating the harms of gentrification to communities of color is a pressing challenge. One promising approach is preference policies that enable long-term residents to remain in or return to gentrifying neighborhoods. This mixed-methods study evaluates the City of Portland's "Preference Policy," which provides targeted affordable rental housing to residents displaced from a historically Black neighborhood. This paper draws on survey, interview, and focus group data to explore resident motivations, changes to well-being, and recommendations for improving the policy. Findings suggest preference policies can enhance well-being, and underscore the need for comprehensive strategies to advance racial justice in gentrifying neighborhoods.

No longer just a problem for a few neighborhoods within the nation's population centers, gentrification is now reaching many small and mid-sized cities (Maciag, 2015; Yonto & Thill, 2020). As a process of neighborhood change, gentrification is generally characterized by a rapid increase in land values and the co-occurring transformation of an area's socioeconomic demographics (Lees et al., 2013). Neighborhoods that are home to communities of color have been particularly vulnerable to and disproportionately harmed by gentrification (as examples, see Gibson, 2007; Li et al., 2013). One of the greatest policy challenges is how to support residents to be able to stay in or return to the neighborhood after it has begun to gentrify.

In response, some cities are experimenting with "right to return" (or community preference) policies that link displaced residents with rental and homeownership opportunities in their former neighborhood (Iglesias, 2018). Racial reparation is at the heart of such policies: they simultaneously acknowledge the harms resulting from historic systemic racism – namely the disruption and displacement of communities of color – and seek to redress those harms through material investments in housing for those displaced, within their historical neighborhoods. If effective, right to return policies advance racial justice by creating housing affordability and stability in gentrifying areas; increase access to neighborhoods that are rich in amenities and resources, particularly for Black residents and other residents of color; and interrupt economic and racial segregation. However, given the limited use and evaluation of these policies to date, there is little evidence regarding if and how right to return policies achieve these aspired goals.

Given that gentrification sits at the intersection of several key challenges identified by the American Academy of Social Work and Social Welfare – including reducing extreme economic inequality, ending homelessness, and eliminating racism – it is critical to innovate, implement and evaluate policy responses to gentrification. This study considers how one of the first community preference policies implemented in a gentrifying neighborhood has advanced racial justice and affected well-being.

Gentrification, community preference policies and community well-being

Gentrification results from a combination of state policy and market response that historically created marginalized, under-resourced areas of communities of color in the urban core, while building exclusionary White neighborhoods for homebuyers in the suburbs (Alfieri, 2019; Massey & Denton, 1993). The disinvestment suppressed land values in many urban neighborhoods, making them vulnerable to gentrification – a sudden influx of capital and new residents taking advantage redevelopment opportunities. A key manifestation of gentrification is the displacement of poor and low-income residents who can no longer afford to remain in place as housing prices rise, accompanied by a changing commercial, institutional, and cultural landscape (Bates, 2013). This displacement has material consequences like housing instability that disrupts schooling and work, and also psycho-social health impacts that social psychiatrist Mindy Fullilove has termed *root shock*. Developed in the context of residents displaced by Urban Renewal, root shock is "the traumatic stress reaction to the loss of some or all of one's emotional ecosystem" (Fullilove, 2016). Displacement due to gentrification threatens the well-being of people, families, and communities when they are involuntarily uprooted.

The consideration of root shock and displacement due to an upward swing in urban neighborhoods is relatively new. For decades, housing policy advocates focused attention on the problems of neighborhood deterioration and concentrated poverty, promoting policies to support low-income people of color to "Move to Opportunity" and tearing down high-density public housing to build mixed-income developments in the HOPE VI program. These policies aimed to de-segregate housing and communities and provide access to place-based opportunity structures, but have had only mixed results for individuals and families (E. G. Goetz, 2010). Now, the dynamic of rapid urban redevelopment has shifted the focus of housing and community development policy. As concerns about displacement due to gentrification have arisen in cities across the U. S., advocates recommended a policy agenda to build and preserve affordable housing within these changing neighborhoods (Kennedy & Leonard, 2001; Levy et al., 2006). Recognizing that once-distressed neighborhoods are now becoming resource-rich with the influx of high-income and mostly White residents, the idea of supporting low-income, renting, and people of color households to stay in place has arisen as an anti-segregation policy.

One promising area of innovation is community preference policies that create affordable housing within the original/former neighborhood for long-term and displaced residents (E. Goetz, 2019; Iglesias, 2018). There have been long-standing resident preference policies in the context of subsidized housing renovation, in which residents have the first claim on redeveloped units. This new use of preference policies addresses the broader context in gentrifying neighborhoods that are changing enough to create re-segregation as people of color are displaced.

Given the degree to which historical and institutionalized racism has led to disparate consequences in housing and access to opportunity for people of color, housing policy leaders increasingly adopt a racial equity lens when considering how best to respond to gentrification (Bates, 2018). Preference policies must thread a careful legal argument to address housing access for people of color, as U.S. Fair Housing and civil rights policy forbid race-specific housing programs, but does allow for mitigation of disparate harms (Alfieri, 2019; Iglesias, 2018). Critics of preference policies express concern that such policies will deepen residential racial and economic segregation (Goodman, 2019). Proponents argue that residents are more likely to access place-based opportunity and resources in their "old" neighborhoods in desirable locations, as well as maintaining their community connections that support well-being (E. Goetz, 2019). There are a growing number of gentrifying cities that have adopted community preference policies (including Seattle, Austin, and San Francisco), combining affordable housing development and preservation with resident prioritization to maintain affordable housing and racial and economic diversity in gentrifying areas (E. Goetz, 2019). This new use of community preference in affordable housing programs offers a window for research about whether a "right to return" to a neighborhood supports access to opportunity and well-being for low-income people of color.

The relationship of gentrification and preference policies to community well-being

Preference policies are designed to be reparative in two ways, first through both the development and siting of affordable housing in gentrifying areas, and second, through the creation of priority access for households that already feel an affinity and have existing networks in the neighborhood. In this way, preference policies are intended to not simply provide housing to but to ameliorate root shock. The individual, family, and community impacts of root shock can be understood through the construct of community well-being.

Wiseman and Brasher define community well-being as "the combination of social, economic, environmental, cultural, and political conditions identified by individuals and their communities as essential for them to flourish and fulfill their potential" (Wiseman & Brasher, 2008, p. 358). Although widely understood as a multidimensional construct, scholars differ on which domains constitute community well-being, and how these domains are operationalized. Measurement of community well-being often contains both objective factors such as housing affordability or amount of green space, and subjective factors such as perceptions of safety and feelings of inclusion (Lee & Kim, 2016; Sung & Phillips, 2016). This paper focuses on four dimensions of well-being: equity and inclusion, social connection, place attachment, and civic participation. The following examples illustrate the potential harms of gentrification to each of these domains, with attention to the disparate effects of gentrification on communities of color. As the effects of preference policies have yet to be studied, we hypothesize the potential effects to well-being for long-term residents who access preference policies to return to or remain in gentrifying neighborhoods.

Equity and inclusion

Black, Latino, and immigrant communities have consistently invested in their own neighborhoods, forming robust business, cultural, and residential districts (Lipsitz, 2011). However, in the face of shifting demographics and upscaling of residential and commercial areas, long-time residents may appear "out of place" in their own neighborhoods and face increased surveillance and policing (Stabrowski, 2014). Long-term residents living in gentrifying areas report increases in racism, classism, and other forms of oppression (Drew, 2012). This causes particular harm in historically Black communities and other ethnic enclaves that function as spaces of support and protection in the face of marginalization from the dominant culture (Drew, 2012). Preference policies have the potential to stem the racialized displacement of long-term residents from gentrifying neighborhoods, which may ensure the area's continued function as a racially "safe space." It is unclear if and how preference policies might reduce racism and other forms of oppression.

Social connection

As neighborhoods gentrify and some residents are priced out, residents may lose access to neighbors and friends they relied on for comradery, social support, and resource sharing (Hodkinson & Essen, 2015; Twigge-Molecey, 2014). This can be particularly damaging in communities of color, where social cohesion can buffer against experiences of racism and other forms of oppression (Hudson, 2015). Preference policies might improve social well-being if returning/remaining residents have, or make, strong social ties in the neighborhood. In the absence of such relationships, returning residents might experience increased isolation and deteriorating social well-being.

Place attachment

Feelings of connection to place contribute to well-being (Plunkett et al., 2018). Gentrification threatens long-term residents' place attachment by erasing historical place names and rebranding neighborhoods to appeal to a wealthier demographic (Hodkinson & Essen, 2015). In such settings, long-term residents may no longer feel comfortable or that they belong (Drew, 2012; Huyser & Meerman, 2014). If residents have strong place-attachments, preference policies may improve their well-being by creating access to stable, affordable housing in the area. However, given spatial transformations within gentrifying neighborhoods, residents might also experience a diminished sense of place attachment.

Civic participation

Gentrification may be accompanied by the political displacement of long-term residents by newer residents who gain control of groups such as neighborhood associations, tenant and homeowner associations, and parent organizations (Davidson, 2008; Freidus, 2019). Without institutional authority, long-term residents have less power to influence decisions that directly affect their neighborhood, or to address legacies of structural racism (Freidus, 2019). Though preference policies do not in and of themselves build power among long-term residents, it is possible that such policies can enhance civic well-being by helping to sustain a robust population of long-term residents who can engage in their communities.

As explored above, gentrification has the potential for widespread adverse effects across multiple domains of well-being; it can disrupt social ties, diminish place attachments, weaken civic engagement, and escalate racism, classism, and other forms of oppression. Most policy responses to gentrification are only designed to address residents' housing needs. By leveraging residents' existing social, spatial, and civic ties, preference policies have the potential to address these other dimensions of well-being that are "essential for [individuals and their communities] to flourish and fulfill their potential" (Wiseman & Brasher, 2008, p. 358). However, the degree to which preference policies can fulfill this potential is unknown. Studying the effects of Portland, Oregon's Preference Policy provides a critical opportunity to understand the policy's impacts on returning residents' well-being, how such policies might be strengthened, and the ways that residents themselves may contribute to the well-being of their communities.

Study context

The study context is in Portland, Oregon, in what the City identifies as the Interstate Corridor Urban Renewal Area (ICURA), known to many residents as the *Albina district*. For more than 60 years, the Albina district in Northeast Portland has served as the residential, economic, spiritual and cultural heart of the city's Black community; over ninety percent of Black Oregonians lived in Albina (Gibson, 2007). The City's designation of multiple Urban Renewal Areas from the 1950s through 2000 in this area resulted in disruptions to the fabric of the neighborhood. In the midcentury, eminent domain was used to build sports stadia and highways; the 2000 ICURA designation extended light rail and spurred further investment. A wave of new boutiques, markets, and restaurants opened, and the resident demographics trended younger, wealthier, and whiter (Gibson, 2007). By 2010, the area lost two-thirds of its Black residents to gentrification and displacement (Bates, 2013). As of 2010, 15% of residents within the ICURA identified as Black, more than twice the city average, but there are no longer any majority-Black Census tracts in Albina (Portland Housing Bureau, 2019). Despite these rapid changes, the Albina district remains a Black cultural center, with multiple Black churches, institutions like the Urban League and the Black United Fund, Oregon's only majority-Black high school, and cultural, art, and entertainment activities focusing on Oregon's Black history.

Perhaps the strongest indicator of the neighborhood's continued significance has been anti-gentrification organizing by the Black community, including making the demand that the City stop displacement and create opportunities for Black families to return to Northeast Portland. In 2015, following the protest of a contentious urban renewal-funded commercial development, the City of Portland adopted a N/NE Housing Strategy with specific rental development, home repair loans and grants, and homeownership goals (Bates, 2018). A key aspect of the strategy is a Preference Policy that prioritizes applicants "who were displaced, are at risk of displacement, or are the descendants of families displaced due to urban renewal in N/NE Portland" (Portland Housing Bureau, 2019, p. 109). Households whose incomes are below 60% of area median income are eligible for priority placement in subsidized, regulated housing units by demonstrating that they, their parents, and/or their grandparents lived within the boundaries of City-drawn urban renewal areas from 1957 to 2000. The policy recognizes generational ties to the community through a point system, with the highest "preference" awarded to those whose residences were taken by eminent domain.

Despite strong community interest in accessing Preference Policy housing, given the degree of gentrification and the resulting loss of economic, social and cultural supports in the neighborhood, it is unclear how the policy will affect well-being. There are three specific aims of this study: (1) *To identify the range of residents' motivations to seek housing through the Preference Policy.* Understanding resident motivation is key to centering the intended beneficiaries in evaluating the effects of the policy. We hypothesize that residents will be motivated by both a need for affordable housing and a desire to live in the N/NE area, and will have expectations regarding both the quality of their housing and their quality of life. (2) *To assess residents' self-reported well-being over time.* As explored above, the well-being literature suggests that the Preference Policy's effects may be mixed; we hypothesize that residents may experience benefits and risks to well-being. (3) *To identify opportunities to strengthen returning residents' well-being.* The Preference Policy was conceptualized as a housing policy. We hypothesize that residents will recommend complementary strategies to improve community well-being. Taken together, these three aims can assist scholars and practitioners in assessing the effectiveness of the policy, guiding ongoing implementation locally, and informing replication.

Methods

This paper reports on the first phase of a longitudinal inquiry of the Preference Policy. The baseline, exploratory data collected in this phase reflects residents' experiences within the first year living in Preference Policy housing, and will serve as comparison data for subsequent rounds of data collection. The majority of the city's $60 million investment has been in rental development, which is the focus of this paper. By the start of 2020, the Portland Housing Bureau had funded the construction of seven apartment buildings containing 531 Preference Policy units, for which there were several thousand applicants (Portland Housing Bureau, 2019).

The study population included all residents living in the first three Preference Policy apartment buildings to open (N = 137). Using a convergent, mixed-method approach (Fetters et al., 2013), the research team sequentially collected surveys (N:98), and conducted interviews (N = 29), and focus groups in each building (28 participants across three groups). After distributing an informational letter to residents, researchers recruited adult participants through door knocking. Participants completed a survey that included questions regarding their motivations for applying to the Preference Policy and a point-in-time assessment of well-being along a number of domains (i.e. sense of community, experience of equity, civic engagement). During the survey, researchers recruited residents to participate in semi-structured interviews, which averaged 30 minutes, and explored residents' relationship to the neighborhood over time, the Preference Policy's impact on their quality of life, and their experiences within the broader neighborhood. After collecting surveys and interviews in each building, researchers hosted a focus group. We shared major findings from their building-level survey data and facilitated a conversation about results and resident's ideas to improve well-being. The focus groups served as an additional source of data collection, a method of participatory analysis, and as a form of member checking.

The response rate for the survey was 69%. At the time of the survey, residents had been living in their new apartments between one and 15 months, averaging 7 months. Participants reported having lived in the Albina District on average for 32 years and 72% of their life. Eighty-four percent of respondents identified as Black or African American, and 68% identified as female. Participant ages ranged between 19–71, with an average age of 43. Most (54%) did not have children living in the home. The majority of apartments were studio or one-bedroom units).

As a *qualitatively-driven inquiry* (Hesse-Biber et al., 2015), this study's focus is to understand residents' motivations, experiences, and perspectives rather than make predictions or determine causation. Researchers analyzed quantitative survey data to identify patterns among respondents, including resident demographics, motivators for applying for the Preference Policy, and reported levels of well-being. All focus groups and interviews were audio-recorded and transcribed, then imported into MaxQDA for analysis. Initial research questions provided an entry point for thematic analysis (Nowell et al., 2017). After Amie Thurber coded a portion of data from each of the three buildings, the coauthors reviewed the initial analysis to check for conceptual clarity, duplicative and missing codes. Thurber then coded the corpus of data. To increase the trustworthiness and credibility of our analysis, we engaged in investigator, methodological, and data triangulation (Lincoln & Guba, 1985; Nowell et al., 2017).

Results

Analysis of data produced three major findings. First, *place matters* deeply to respondents; residents were motivated to apply for the Preference Policy by both the location and the cost of housing. Second, residents report experiencing overall *improved well-being* since moving into their units. And third, residents also report some *threats to well-being*, particularly related to economic vulnerability and the persistence of racism.

Place matters

Understanding residents' motivations for applying to the Preference Policy is necessary to evaluate one of the policy's central assumptions: that the location, as well as the affordability, of housing matters to renters. This assumption proved largely correct: 80% of respondents indicated that both feeling a connection to the neighborhood *and* a need for housing were primary motivations for applying for housing through the Preference Policy.

Despite the demographic changes in the Albina district, 83% of residents reported having friends and family in the neighborhood, and nearly two-thirds of residents indicated that being closer to those existing social ties was a primary motivation for applying to the Preference Policy. In addition to wanting to be closer to friends and family, many communicated a desire to live in an area with a robust Black community, as reflected by another Black woman resident who concluded: "There's nothing wrong with wanting to be around my people." Spatial aspects of the neighborhood – such as local organizations, businesses, parks, and schools – also mattered to many residents. More than 70% of those surveyed indicated that being "closer to the places I like to go" was a primary motivation for applying for Preference Policy housing. Many of the specific places named were culturally significant to residents, such as Dawson Park, a historic gathering spot for Black civic events. A sense of connection to the neighborhood over time also mattered to participants. Nine out of ten respondents agreed with the statement, "the history of this neighborhood matters to me." In interviews, many residents traced their family history in the area, sometimes over generations. Several residents described their family's migration from the south, seeking work in Portland's shipyards, and settling in the Albina district. A resident in her 20s proudly shared that her great-grandmother has owned her home in the neighborhood since 1930. Participants broadly shared this feeling of comfort and belonging; 87% agreed with the statement, "I belong in this neighborhood."

Importantly, residents were equally motivated by a need for affordable housing. Though the survey did not directly ask if residents had been previously homeless, 10% of respondents volunteered that they were unhoused prior to moving into their new apartment. Eighty percent believed that the Preference Policy was their best chance to move from a waitlist into housing, and nearly sixty percent indicated this was their only real housing option. As a formerly homeless Black resident put it, "I did want to stay in this area. But I had to find something that fit my budget." The Preference Policy buildings made achieving these twin goals possible.

It is noteworthy that a small number of respondents were *not* motivated by feelings of connection to the neighborhood; this was most frequently described by people who had lived in the area only briefly. For the vast majority of respondents, residents' deep social and spatial attachments to the Albina district – combined with a need for affordable housing – motivated them to apply to the Preference Policy, and they carried the expectation that the policy would not only address their housing needs, but help them achieve other dimensions of well-being.

Improved well-being

Overwhelmingly, residents reported improvements to community well-being since accessing housing through the Preference Policy, particularly related to equity and inclusion, social connection, place attachment, and civic engagement. Although the following sections explore these themes independently, in practice, they were often interrelated.

Equity and inclusion

Many expressed appreciation for living in a neighborhood where they experience lower levels of prejudice than elsewhere in the city. Seventy percent of those surveyed agreed that people of different backgrounds get along in the neighborhood. A number of those interviewed contrasted living in the Albina district to other areas of Portland that are less racially diverse, particularly suburbs that had been destinations for "white flight" in previous decades. Regarding her move, a Black mother living with her school-aged child reflected:

> ... it's improved my quality of life because I'm not as stressed out. My neighborhood in Gresham [a Portland suburb] was way worse. It was very White out there, and ... There was a lot of racism out there, and I didn't feel accepted out there, and being back in the neighborhood, I'm glad this building is predominantly Black. I can feel comfortable around Black people, and if anything, it's improved my quality of life.

As evidenced above, the experiences of equity and area demographics were intimately tied: many residents reported experiencing less racism living in areas with a larger Black population.

Social connection

Most of those interviewed noted the social benefits of living where they have existing social connections and also feel a broader sense of community. When asked what it felt like to return to the neighborhood, a Black mother who grew up in the neighborhood explained, "Kind of a relief, like a sigh in a way. It just felt comforting to move back to somewhere that- where I've- I know. It's just so close to my family and my friends I grew up with. It's just a really big deal." This theme was echoed in most interviews and focus groups. As a Black grandmother who lived her entire life in N/NE explained, "It's a lot of people that still stay in this neighborhood that I grew up with ... A lot of people still here on the same block." In addition to the benefits of living closer to existing social networks, many residents spoke to the broader social value of living in a robust Black community. One mother explained the importance she placed in moving her daughter out of a predominantly White school: "I wanted her to be able to see the representation. To be around people that look like her, and to not feel like she was so different. It was so important for me to get back on this side of town, for her."

Strikingly, some residents noted that the Preference Policy was helping to stabilize and rebuild the Black community in the area. As one Black mother explained,

The people that grew up in the area, they got moved out and the houses were bought out and all of that. They tore them down, redid them, but I guess they're doing these new developments to try to get people back and it's working. I feel like it's working.

Another resident who lived most of her life in the neighborhood reflected that since the two Preference Policy buildings have opened in her area, "I've actually seen a lot more colored faces, more urban people come back, which is nice. It is really nice." Overwhelmingly, residents expressed improvements in social wellbeing as a result of the Preference Policy.

Place attachment

Respondents voiced nearly universal appreciation for the convenience of living in the neighborhood. Several respondents specifically noted the Black-owned stores in the area, as well as the value of living closer to their church, children's school, Black civic and youth-serving programs, and preferred beauty supply stores and salons. A number of people shared that though they had previously moved out of the Albina district to access more affordable housing, they were still commuting to the neighborhood regularly for community activities. One father of five explained he had moved his family to a suburb, "and we was never there because all of our kids' activities was in Portland . . . I'm not paying $110.00 in gas a week now. It's barely $20.00 a week now for gas." Living closer to the culturally-specific resources and amenities within the Albina district has economic, cultural, and community benefits for Black residents, and has strengthened many resident's place attachments.

Civic participation

Also noteworthy were residents' self-reported increases in civic engagement. Fifty-six percent of residents reported they spend time volunteering regularly – which is significantly higher than the U.S. average of 25% (Bureau of Labor Statistics, 2016) – and a quarter of residents reported that their civic engagement has *increased* since moving into the building. Similarly, 80% of residents reported regularly participating in arts and cultural events, and more than 50% indicated their participation had *increased* since moving into housing. In interviews, many residents credited this increase in civic and cultural engagement to proximity, particularly to Black churches, schools, and civic organizations.

In summary, most respondents identified positive changes in their life as a result of moving into Preference Policy housing: they report greater feelings of equity and inclusion in the Albina district than in other areas of Portland, feel a stronger sense of community and belonging, are closer to the places they want to go, and are more involved in their community. However, as described below, many residents also described threats to their well-being, and the Preference Policy seems to be serving some residents better than others.

Threats to well-being

Though the majority of residents felt their lives improved since moving into Preference Policy housing, many still identified vulnerabilities to their well-being. The two most prevalent areas of risk relate to equity and inclusion: inequitable access to resources and services, and the persistence of racism and other forms of oppression. These were also the two areas where residents had the greatest number of recommendations for neighborhood improvements.

Insufficient access to needed resources and services

Although all Preference Policy units are designated "affordable," a few residents remain very precariously housed. For example, one man in his 60s whose only income is a monthly SSI check of less than $800 reported paying more than $700 each month for rent. Three interviewees shared serious concerns about how they will be able to stay housed. While only a few respondents reported extreme precarity, many reported persistent economic vulnerability that was exacerbated by insufficient affordable stores and shops in the neighborhood, as well as the scarcity of employment opportunities.

When surveyed, residents confirmed that there were many restaurants and stores in the area. Yet, it became evident in interviews and focus groups that many residents did not frequent area businesses. One woman who lived in the neighborhood for about ten years explained, "[I wish there were] more, different stores. Because the stores are so expensive that they put in this area." A third of those interviewed recommended co-locating a low-cost grocery close by their apartment building. The need for jobs was also a concern. Less than half of those surveyed believed that people who want to find a good job in the neighborhood can do so, and several people identified the need for job training programs for young people. Others, like a Black father who grew up in the neighborhood, spoke about the need to invest in more Black-owned businesses: "That will need to come back, and [the city] will have to give the opportunities for Blacks and help Blacks." As demonstrated in this quote, some residents expect the Preference Policy to be accompanied by targeted economic development. In addition, nearly half of those interviewed expressed concern for more affordable rental and homeownership opportunities.

Persistence of racism

Although many residents reported feeling more racially comfortable in the Albina District than in other neighborhoods, residents also reported uneven experiences in this domain. For example, while most agreed that people of different backgrounds get along, 37% also agreed that there's "a lot" of prejudice in the neighborhood, and 30% of those surveyed indicated that they had experienced discrimination in area businesses. The interviews surfaced many examples of marginalization, surveillance, and presumed criminality of Black residents by White neighbors. One gentleman in his 60s shared this example:

> I was carrying a ladder, and I borrowed it from a friend, and this guy came out of his house and had his phone, and he's recording me walking down the street. He walked with me about five blocks, came in front of my house, and filmed me. I said, "Man, what is up with this? I'm not stealing the ladder; it's my friend's ladder. I've got to work on the house, I'm painting . . .

Several recounted experiences of discrimination at area parks that have been long-standing gathering places for Black residents. Residents described White families pulling their children away from playing with residents' children and younger relatives, and being looked at by White people as if they were, in the words of one previously unhoused woman, "an eyesore." As another woman explained, "You walk around, and there's just all White people and they look at you like you ain't supposed to be here. No, *you're* not supposed to be here. I grew up over here . . . " For many, these experiences of racism were particularly hurtful *because* they occurred in an area where residents have deep personal ties and expect to feel racially comfortable more of the time.

The most frequent hope for the neighborhood – shared by nearly 40% of those interviewed – was for greater community cohesion, both within the Black community and across group lines. Many people mentioned events that draw out the Black community each year, such as "Good in the Hood," a day-long street festival, and expressed a desire for more frequent events such as these to nurture Portland's Black community. Several expressed a desire to see more Black families return to the area. As one Black mother with multi-generational history in N/NE explained, she hopes the neighborhood will:

> . . . get back to normal, like how it used to be like. More Blacks in the area, coming back to where they are from and where they grew up. And everybody being able to intertwine. It don't have to be just Black people, but I want people who are not minorities to be able to interact with minorities.

A number of interviewees echoed this desire for non-Black residents to have the ability to interact respectfully across group lines.

Others spoke to the need for intercultural gatherings to build relationships and comfort in the neighborhood. One Black woman in her 30s reflected that her experiences with racism have made her cautious with White people, offering, "I think there needs to be more opportunity to get together and really get together ... personally, I would like to see more opportunities for more intentional gatherings of people." Residents expressed interest in fostering greater community cohesion at various scales, from Sunday potlucks in their building, to block parties designed to build relationships with immediate neighbors, to broader social, cultural, and civic activities.

In summary, though most residents feel that their lives are improving due to having stable, affordable housing through the Preference Policy, insufficient access to needed resources and services, as well as experiences of racism and other forms of oppression, are threats to well-being. As noted above, residents identified a number of complementary economic development and community building strategies to address these areas of concern.

Discussion

The City of Portland is among the first to adopt a place-based preference policy to redress the harms caused to a historically Black neighborhood by past land-use policies and present-day gentrification, and this study is among the first to examine the impacts of such policies on well-being. Results from this first phase of study offer several promising findings. The N/NE Preference Policy has contributed to housing affordability and stability in a gentrifying area, particularly for Black residents with intergenerational ties to the Albina district. Findings also confirmed what the Black community organizers who advocated for the policy knew to be true – that place matters deeply to many of the Albina district's longtime residents. The levels of place attachment reflected in this sample far exceed the national averages. Whereas less than 20% of adults in the U.S. report a strong emotional connection to their community (Carman et al., 2019), the vast majority of respondents in this study expressed particularly strong social connections, place attachments, and above-average levels of civic engagement. By facilitating these residents' ability to live in an area where they already feel connected and are engaged, the Preference Policy contributes to their well-being. Findings imply a secondary benefit as well: the policy may contribute to the broader community's well-being through these returning residents' connection and engagement. In this way, the Preference Policy leverages two important resources to improve community well-being: affordable housing and the residents themselves.

These preliminary findings also suggest limitations of the Preference Policy. Although the policy successfully increases affordable housing in an increasingly desirable neighborhood, residents also need affordable stores and family-supporting jobs. Results underscore that simply *residing* in a neighborhood with abundant amenities does not produce a universal benefit. Furthermore, although the policy approaches reparation for the harms of past policies on residents of a historically Black neighborhood, the policy does not account for persistent racism that shapes residents' experiences living in the neighborhood, or address their desire to strengthen social ties and address intergroup bias. Informed by resident recommendations for economic development and community building, we wonder what it would look like for this policy to be reimagined from a housing strategy to a comprehensive community development strategy that includes attention to housing, jobs, and the civic/social/cultural life of the neighborhood. A holistic strategy imagined and implemented in partnership with government, nonprofit, and civic organizations, can more effectively support the longtime Albina district residents returning to the neighborhood, as well as those who never left.

Thoroughly assessing changes to community well-being requires a longitudinal analysis. In the next phase of this study, the research team will gather data from residents up to three years into their residence in Preference Policy housing, and compare that to the well-being of similar residents residing in other types of neighborhoods. While this study focuses on the policy's effects on those served, a more comprehensive evaluation of the policy is needed to fully consider its effectiveness, particularly toward meeting racial justice goals. Given the policy's reparative aspirations, it is important to ask whether the scale of investment from the City is commensurate to the losses incurred by the Black community, and to consider perspectives of those who have not been served by the policy (such as those who remain on the waitlist and those who did not meet renter eligibility requirements), as well as existing Albina residents.

Conclusion

This study suggests that preference policies can be a critical tool for advancing racial justice and well-being in gentrifying neighborhoods by (1) recognizing the disparate harms of urban development on communities of color; (2) siting affordable housing in areas with existing social, cultural and civic networks; and (3) leveraging the power of returning residents to help rebuild community well-being. In providing insight into how returning residents' well-being is affected positively and negatively by accessing housing in a gentrifying neighborhood to which they have strong ties, the results of this study can inform policies in other contexts where changing neighborhoods have disrupted housing stability. As similar policies are adopted, additional research will be critical to understanding the conditions in which preference policies are more and less effective, and the long-term effects on area demographics and well-being.

Community preference policies are not intended to address all of the harms caused by gentrification. That said, this study suggests preference policies can be an important tool for addressing the disproportionate effects of gentrification on Black communities and other communities of color that have long-standing ties to now-revitalized neighborhoods. However, given the widespread harms of gentrification across multiple domains of well-being, simply increasing affordable housing in gentrifying neighborhoods is insufficient. Advancing racial justice and well-being in gentrifying neighborhoods will require comprehensive community development, including community-engaged assessment of needs and policies and programs that respond to residents' desires for their community. In the context of historic and ongoing systemic racism that continues to shape neighborhood well-being, it will take a holistic approach to rebuild what has been lost and restore a sense of community that will last.

Disclosure statement

No potential conflict of interest was reported by the author(s).

Funding

This work was supported by the Portland State University [2019 Faculty Development Grant, Vision 2025 Seed Data].

ORCID

Amie Thurber ⓘ http://orcid.org/0000-0003-0753-5895
Lisa K. Bates ⓘ http://orcid.org/0000-0002-3887-8754

References

Alfieri, A. V. (2019). Black, poor, and gone: Civil rights law's inner-city crisis. *Harvard Civil Rights-Civil Liberties Law Review*, 54 (2) , 629–702. https://harvardcrcl.org/wp-content/uploads/sites/10/2019/07/54.2-Alfieri.pdf

Bates, L. K. (2013). Gentrification and displacement study: Implementing an equitable inclusive development strategy in the context of gentrification. *City of Portland Bureau of Planning and Sustainability* 1–96 . https://doi.org/10.15760/report-01

Bates, L. K. (2018). Growth without displacement: A test for equity planning in Portland. In N. Krumholz & K. Wertheim Hexter (Eds.), *Advancing equity planning now* (pp. 21–43). Cornell University Press.

Bureau of Labor Statistics. (2016). *Volunteering in the United States — 2015 [press release]*. U.S. Department of Labor. https://www.bls.gov/news.release/pdf/volun.pdf

Carman, K. G., Chandra, A., Weilant, S., Miller, C., & Tait, M. (2019). *2018 national survey of health attitudes: Description and top-line summary data*. RAND. https://www.rand.org/pubs/research_reports/RR2876.html

Davidson, M. (2008). Spoiled mixture: Where does state-led 'positive' gentrification end? *Urban Studies*, 45(12), 2385–2405. https://doi.org/10.1177/0042098008097105

Drew, E. M. (2012). "Listening through white ears": Cross-racial dialogues as a strategy to address the racial effects of gentrification. *Journal of Urban Affairs*, 34(1), 99–115. https://doi.org/10.1111/j.1467-9906.2011.00572.x

Fetters, M. D., Curry, L. A., & Creswell, J. W. (2013). Achieving integration in mixed methods designs—principles and practices. *Health Services Research*, 48(6pt2), 2134–2156. https://doi.org/10.1111/1475-6773.12117

Freidus, A. (2019). "A great school benefits us all": Advantaged parents and the gentrification of an urban public school. *Urban Education*, 54(8), 1121–1148. https://doi.org/10.1177/0042085916636656

Fullilove, M. (2016). *Root shock: How tearing up city neighborhoods hurts America, and what we can do about it*. New Village Press.

Gibson, K. J. (2007). Bleeding Albina: A history of community disinvestment, 1940-2000. *Transforming Anthropology*, 15(1), 3–25. https://doi.org/10.1525/tran.2007.15.1.03

Goetz, E. G. (2010). Desegregation in 3D: Displacement, dispersal and development in American public housing. *Housing Studies*, 25(2), 137–158. https://doi.org/10.1080/02673030903561800

Goetz, E. (2019). *Criticism about community preference policies are misguided*. Shelterforce. https://shelterforce.org/2019/11/14/criticisms-about-community-preference-policies-are-misguided/

Goodman, J. D. (2019, July 16). *What the city didn't want the public to know: Its policy deepens segregation*. The New York Times. https://www.nytimes.com/2019/07/16/nyregion/segregation-nyc-affordable-housing.html

Hesse-Biber, S. N., Bailey-Rodriguez, D., & Frost, N. (2015). A qualitatively driven approach to multimethod and mixed methods research. In S. N. Hesse-Biber & R. B. Johnson (Eds.), *The Oxford handbook of multimethod and mixed methods research inquiry* (pp. 3–20). Oxford University Press.

Hodkinson, S., & Essen, C. (2015). Grounding accumulation by dispossession in everyday life: The unjust geographies of urban regeneration under the private finance initiative. *International Journal of Law in the Built Environment*, 7(1), 72–91. https://doi.org/10.1108/IJLBE-01-2014-0007

Hudson, K. D. (2015). Toward a conceptual framework for understanding community belonging and well-being: Insights from a queer-mixed perspective. *Journal of Community Practice*, 23(1), 27–50. https://doi.org/10.1080/10705422.2014.986595

Huyser, M., & Meerman, J. R. (2014). Resident perceptions of redevelopment and gentrification in the heartside neighborhood: Lessons for social work profession. *Journal of Sociology & Social Welfare*, 41(3), 3–22. https://scholarworks.wmich.edu/jssw/vol41/iss3/2

Iglesias, T. (2018). Threading the needle of fair housing law in a gentrifying city with a legacy of discrimination. *Journal of Affordable Housing & Community Development*, 27(1), 51–65. https://link.gale.com/apps/doc/A568258468/AONE?u=s1185784&sid=bookmark-AONE&xid=fbb6cb06

Kennedy, M., & Leonard, P. (2001). *Dealing with neighborhood change: A primer on gentrification and policy choices*. Brookings Institution Center on Urban and Metropolitan Policy. https://www.brookings.edu/research/dealing-with-neighborhood-change-a-primer-on-gentrification-and-policy-choices/

Lee, S. J., & Kim, Y. (2016). Structure of well-being: An exploratory study of the distinction between individual well-being and community well-being and the importance of intersubjective community well-being. In Y. Kee, S. Lee, & R. Phillips (Eds.), *Social factors and community well-being* (pp. 13–37). Springer.

Lees, L., Slater, T., & Wyly, E. (2013). *Gentrification*. Routledge.

Levy, D. K., Comey, J., & Padilla, S. (2006). *In the face of gentrification: Case studies of local efforts to mitigate displacement*. The Urban Institute. https://www.urban.org/sites/default/files/publication/50791/411294-In-the-Face-of-Gentrification.PDF

Li, B. Y., Vitiello, D., & Acoca, A. (2013). *Chinatown then and now: Gentrification in Boston, New York and Philadelphia*. Asian American Legal Defense and Education Fund. http://aaldef.org/Chinatown%20Then%20and%20Now%20AALDEF.pdf

Lincoln, Y., & Guba, E. (1985). *Naturalistic inquiry*. Sage.

Lipsitz, G. (2011). *How racism takes place*. Temple University Press.

Maciag, M. (2015). *Gentrification in America report*. Governing. http://www.governing.com/gov-data/census/gentrification-in-cities-governing-report.html

Massey, D., & Denton, N. A. (1993). *American apartheid: Segregation and the making of the underclass*. Harvard University Press.

Nowell, L. S., Norris, J. M., White, D. E., & Moules, N. J. (2017). Thematic analysis: Striving to meet the trustworthiness criteria. *International Journal of Qualitative Methods*, 16(1), 1609406917733847. https://doi.org/10.1177/1609406917733847

Plunkett, D., Phillips, R., & Ucar Kocaoglu, B. (2018). Place attachment and community development. *Journal of Community Practice*, 26(4), 471–482. https://doi.org/10.1080/10705422.2018.1521352

Portland Housing Bureau. (2019). *State of housing in Portland*. https://www.portland.gov/sites/default/files/2020-04/phb-soh-2019-web.pdf

Stabrowski, F. (2014). New-build gentrification and the everyday displacement of Polish immigrant tenants in Greenpoint, Brooklyn. *Antipode*, 46(3), 794–815. https://doi.org/10.1111/anti.12074

Sung, H., & Phillips, R. (2016). Conceptualizing a community well-being and theory construct. In Y. Kee, S. J. Lee, & R. Phillips (Eds.), *Social factors and community well-being* (pp. 1–12). Springer.

Twigge-Molecey, A. (2014). Exploring resident experiences of indirect displacement in a neighbourhood undergoing gentrification: The case of Saint-Henri in Montreal. *Canadian Journal of Urban Research*, 23(1), 1–22. https://link.gale.com/apps/doc/A398951168/AONE?u=oregon_oweb&sid=googleScholar&xid=4fb8903a

Wiseman, J., & Brasher, K. (2008). Community wellbeing in an unwell world: Trends, challenges, and possibilities. *Journal of Public Health Policy*, 29(3), 353–366. https://doi.org/10.1057/jphp.2008.16

Yonto, D., & Thill, J. C. (2020). Gentrification in the US New South: Evidence from two types of African American communities in Charlotte. *Cities*, 97, 102475. https://doi.org/10.1016/j.cities.2019.102475

Minority Political Leadership Institute: a model for developing racial equity leadership

Nakeina E. Douglas-Glenn [iD], Shabana K. Shaheen, Elizabeth P. Marlowe, and Kiara S. Faulks

ABSTRACT
Building leadership capacity centered on the interests and needs of racial and ethnic minoritized communities is critical and complex. This exploratory qualitative case study examined the Minority Political Leadership Institute and its novel approach to developing racial equity leaders in a community context. The findings outline the effective strategies used to engage participants and communities and provide insight into the lessons learned in program design and delivery.

Designing effective programs to increase leadership capacity is complex. Stakes are higher when programs address race-related societal pressures. Unfortunately, most connections between race and leadership largely occur outside of leadership studies (Dugan, 2017; Furman, 2012; Ospina & Foldy, 2009). Whereas references to social justice are abundant, race is highlighted among many other diversity factors, given little analytical legitimacy, or left on the margins of the leadership discourse (Ospina & Foldy, 2009).

Leadership development programs offer a means to mitigate these concerns by combining skill development with raised consciousness (Day & Harrison, 2007). Leadership programs go beyond the transfer of knowledge and individual skill acquisition (leader development), emphasizing insight on one's relationship to others and building collective capacity (leadership development) (Stech, 2008; Van De Valk, 2008). In this instance, leadership is motivated by efforts to redress structural inequity built into rules that govern society (Ospina, 2017 by linking leader development with social phenomena to help people understand how to collaborate, build relationships and commitments, and develop extended social networks within broader social systems (Curral et al., 2016).

This article reflects on the Minority Political Leadership Institute (MPLI) as a novel approach for building the capacity of racial and ethnic group leaders in Virginia's political and civic landscape. This examination considers the pivotal program components and deliberates the implications and utility of MPLI as a community leadership development program model for promoting anti-racist work.

Theoretical framework

Critical theories are appropriate for engaging race as a social justice issue in leadership (Gooden & Dantley, 2012). Critical Race Theory (CRT) applies a critical interrogation of leadership definitions, practices, and contexts that have reinforced racial inequity. CRT yields insights into power relations, social processes, and patterns of oppression and domination within leadership (Chandler & Kirsch, 2018). A race-conscious framework, CRT posits race and racism are situated in all human conditions; race is socially constructed; race advantages the interests of whites; voices of the marginalized should be elevated; and intersecting oppression exists (Delgado et al., 2001).

Leadership development programs fail when they neglect to focus on the context in which leadership occurs (Gurdjian et al., 2014). Black and Brown leaders have been disadvantaged by a prevailing leadership environment that has primarily excluded their participation. White, high-income, and highly educated professionals have typically occupied community leadership programs giving moderate attention to diversity (Valdes, 2001). MPLI is committed to reversing this impediment by transforming leadership in the political arena. Situating Black and Brown leaders and communities at the forefront of leadership development offers a counter-narrative to the dominant standard of leadership as white (Carton & Rosette, 2011; Haynie, 2002; Rosette et al., 2008) and public policy without racial consequence (Saito, 2009). MPLI challenges prevailing leadership narratives by emphasizing outcomes deeply rooted in the historical and contemporary structural situation of Black and Brown communities. A structural view of race helps analyze the culmination of practices and institutional arrangements that have co-created racial inequality (powell, 2013). Acknowledging structural racialization advances an interpretation of society's origination through a racial lens (Bonilla-Silva, 1997).

Methods

This study uses a single case study approach to describe and analyze MPLI. This approach allows deep insights into the how, what, and why of a phenomenon within a particular context (Evers & Wu, 2006; Patton, 2015; Yin, 2018). Qualitative case studies are an extensive part of the business, management, and leadership literature mainly because of their flexibility and suitability for capturing social phenomena (Halkias & Neubert, 2020). This study identified and documented the effective strategies for engaging leaders to promote racial equity; descriptions of participant experiences before, during, and after participation; and lessons learned about social justice, racial equity, and leadership. Data were collected from archival records and focus groups with program alumni, for which approval from the Institutional Review Board was received. Data collection from different evidence sources ensures rigor in the study design and construct validity (Yin, 2018). Two lead researchers facilitated the focus groups via Zoom, which were recorded with permission. Each focus group lasted approximately 90 minutes.

Sample

Focus group participants were recruited using the program's alumni listserv and included 13 participants from cohorts between 2012 and 2018. Study participants represented five employment sectors: higher education, corporate, nonprofit, public agencies, and faith-based. Almost two-thirds of the participants identified as Black/African American (64.3%); 14% identified as Asian, 7% as American Indian/Alaska Native, and 14% as white.

Data analysis

Thematic analysis included organizing the derived data into themes (Creswell & Creswell, 2017). Archival records, including participant applications, program syllabi, session evaluations, and pre- and post-assessments provided historical accounts of MPLI's operations. Participants' perspectives captured from focus group discussions provided additional data. Focus group transcriptions were checked for accuracy following each session and independently coded by the authors to classify and interpret the findings using an iterative process to draw conclusions (Evers & Wu, 2006).

The case: the Minority Political Leadership Institute

Context

Since its inception, MPLI has emerged as a premier resource in Virginia for developing leaders of color (Wilson, 2017) committed to addressing minoritized communities' policy needs. Administered against the legacy of the "Virginia Way," MPLI entered a leadership development arena already occupied by prominent regional programs that afforded marginal attention to the needs of Black leaders or their communities. Virginia's long-held corporate-centric philosophy strategically structured social and political life around paternalism and power, with whites maintaining considerable economic, political, and social control (Smith, 2002; Thomas, 2019). With very real consequences for racial and ethnic minoritized groups, the Virginia Way did not see Black people as capable of self-determination, locking them out of policy and governance except when it suited white rule (Constable, 2021). Members of the Virginia Legislative Black Caucus (VLBC) and program faculty believed MPLI to be a vehicle for promoting Black self-determination for community issues with the aim of creating political leaders to counterpose the heavily white commanding rule.

Vision and mission

MPLI is best characterized as a community leadership development program focused on the leader and leadership development of early and mid-career professionals at the intersection of race and policy/politics. The program's curriculum is built around four priorities: racial equity, leadership presence, capacity building, and collaborative leadership. These combine individual learning with shared experience to shift the balance of political influence. Shared learning between leaders within the program and those across the community builds the bench of diverse leaders across the state with knowledge, capabilities, and access to increase their influence on behalf of greater minoritized community outcomes.

MPLI is a biennial, eight-month experience. Participants meet for two days a month, and program faculty and external consultants provide instruction. Members of the VLBC, other supportive political figures, well-renowned leaders, and relevant authorities from the community, state, and national arenas provide inspiration and practical guidance. In 2012, the program made significant changes to include Latinx and Native American communities, given their shared experiences of exclusion, disadvantage, and barriers to opportunity (Enchautegui, 2015) with Black/African American communities in Virginia (Khine, 2019). Although some sessions are annually altered (based on the changing policy landscape, competitive environment, and emerging best practices), the curriculum framework remains stable.

Participants

Between 20 and 25 participants are invited to participate each year. Since 2004, 176 people have participated. Of the 176 program participants, more than half (84%) self-identified as Black/African American. Women comprised over 60% of all participants. Historically, the program has attracted individuals with diverse professional backgrounds, including credentialed, educational, service, and independent professionals. Most participants (51%) were public sector employees. Civic interests and engagement among participants were vast;

more than half reported involvement in community or civic organizations (75%), volunteering with campaigns (50%), and future interests in state and local boards and commissions (56%).

Signature features of the program

MPLI is designed to disrupt the existing networks of politics, opening access to political leadership platforms from which they have been otherwise locked out. It helps participants decode access and opportunity to leadership in the political and policy arenas.

Leader and leadership development

MPLI focuses on both leader and leadership development in its curriculum design and delivery (Porr, 2011). A scaffolded approach is employed to advance individual efficacy (Bandura, 1997; Murphy & Ensher, 1999; Paglis & Green, 2002) through developmental assignments, retrospective and prospective reflections, and personal assessments. Attention to leader self-efficacy is then tied to collective efficacy (Bandura, 1997; Hannah et al., 2008) through team development activities, site visits, action-based learning, state-wide travel, and community networking. Through these complementary and integrated experiences, participants begin to develop a collective approach to their leadership with other program participants, the communities encountered, and the areas they serve. By the end of this experience, participants possess a greater belief in the group's common ability and capacity to produce a change in racial equity.

State-wide immersion

MPLI relies on an orientation strategy (Azzam & Riggio, 2003) whereby participants are moved out of their comfort zone to understand community (Dudziak & Profitt, 2012; Weng & Clark, 2017). Each program cycle begins in central Virginia. From there, participants travel to five major regions in the state and learn from the life experiences and community voices in the geographical and cultural context. Experiential knowledge is garnered from firsthand accounts of community members and leaders about policy issues and trends, thus validating and challenging racism (Christian et al., 2019). As one participant described, "The ability to hear firsthand how government and social structures affected the lives of people. . . . . it's important to understand the whole history." Understanding social justice as community insiders minimizes the risk of engaging in policy-making and service delivery methods that perpetuate injustice (Weng & Clark, 2017).

Racial equity analysis of legislation

Participants examine the racial impact of legislation through project-based learning. Conducting legislative racial equity analysis is essential for examining public policy effects on minoritized communities and exposing claims of race neutrality. Its purpose is two-fold: (1) it examines how specific legislation promotes or reduces racial/ethnic disparities for minoritized communities; and (2) the experience of conducting an analysis develops a cadre of leaders who focus on racial equity, which is a vital skill set to achieve better outcomes for communities of color. A participant explained, "The biggest thing is just being able to define it. I [have] gained the words, the ideas, and the data, to define it and deal with it." Throughout the process, participants engage with key stakeholders, research problems, and define solutions. Through these experiential learning opportunities, participants advance their knowledge of racial equity in ways that connect theory and research in their leadership practice:

> what the program made me realize is the power in the data ... They tell a story that supports the argument of social injustice or social inequity. That helps us push for better policy and better changes in the law ... when we did the research ... that was mind blowing, for me ...

Participants advance what they learned and its relevance to racial equity through a capstone presentation locally and nationally.

Participant reflections

Overall, participants reported greater clarity in their leadership vision for social justice after program participation and a substantive increase in knowledge and awareness in four key areas: general and legislative issues affecting underserved communities in Virginia, awareness of the historical influence on issues that remain unaddressed, and awareness of social equity approaches used to promote racial equity. They also reported increased expertise in building a climate of inclusion, promoting solutions for underserved communities' issues, and their ability to perform as a results-oriented change agent in organizational settings and community-based endeavors. Participants reported their values, beliefs, opinions, and expectations regarding social justice, racial equity, and leadership were based on their personal experiences before the program.

Social justice

For several participants, mainly social workers and legislative aides, the program validated their social justice perspectives rather than leading to a shift in their paradigms. Enhanced citizenry was viewed as essential to fortifying equity for the next generation. MPLI was viewed as "an opportunity for us to look at how we send a rope back down to help folks, and ... remove some of these structural barriers to promote equity and equality." One participant reflected that the program allowed them to speak about expansive community development. Participants discussed a shift from their individualized conceptualization of social justice to a more communal definition and understanding. Consistent with findings from Bono et al. (2010) participants were motivated to be more intentionally additive, personally and professionally, by leveraging themselves to create potential, opportunity, and sustainable infrastructure for others: "We're building communities; we're creating a sense of racial equity in these communities. That is going to be there for years and decades to come."

Racial equity

Overall, participants felt participation bolstered their prior beliefs about racial equity. Participants remarked that lessons about the structural saturation of race outlined in the program significantly contributed to how they perceived contemporary issues. Following the program, participants described themselves as "racial equity prepared" on two fronts. First, they could identify matters of racial equity with greater clarity and confidence. Second, they were better able to apply a racial equity framework to their personal and professional experiences. Several themes, including the damaging effects of Jim Crow, mass incarceration, limited educational opportunities, housing insecurity, and extreme poverty, were examined differently after the program. Hearing firsthand accounts of racial injustice led to a more humanized understanding of the legacy of structural barriers. For example, one participant reflected on their experience after a visit to the Robert Russa Moton Museum, a school site where former students tell their stories about massive resistance in Virginia: " ... seeing the school and seeing where it actually happened. And what the conditions were. I mean, it just, it moves you." The experience provided them with greater capacity to mitigate circumstances created from a system of inequity. MPLI participants incorporate a new vision of racial equity into their professional practice and apply the program's tools to their roles.

Leadership

Participants reported a shift in their views on leadership. There was increased desire for more extraordinary personal leadership. For those with experience in politics, MPLI was effective to overcome the leadership deficits in their profession. MPLI affirmed their perspective that leaders beneficial for their communities can be developed (Fredericks, 2003). The program empowered participants to view themselves as qualified leaders who could occupy a similar space as elected leaders and initiate racial equity conversations, "going through the program has given me a totally different perspective on what I can lead in my own space. I don't have to be elected to office in order to lead or to do what I need to do ... to impact ... any kind of change." Participants reflected on the program's preparation and impact on their transition to higher professional positions. They provided examples of using their professional capacity "to more effectively and strategically deal with and even combat some of the things that have created a system of inequity" in service provision, policy implementation, and new political appointments. Transformations in leadership approach and style were identified. Tools and language acquisition allowed for more significant community organizing; shared understanding and language expedited the ability to focus on the communities' issues.

After completing the program, participants reported a paradigm shift. They left MPLI motivated to pursue additional personal development opportunities, training, and education in racial equity. Another significant theme was building and sustaining relationships. The opportunity to connect and share personal stories with other program participants and the people they met during their travels across the state was substantial. Relationships were seen as pivotal to achieving racial equity goals. The experience helped them appreciate their relationship with the greater community.

Implications for community practice

This case study demonstrates a dynamic paradigm for leadership development that advances racial equity. It adds to the literature an understanding of what works in community (Fredericks, 1999) and civic (Azzam & Riggio, 2003) leadership programs. MPLI's success is primarily due to its ability to produce a community leadership development program that focuses on leader and leadership development at the intersection of race and policy/politics. MPLI creates a liberatory space (Waite, 2021) for participants to freely engage and consider race as a central operating function of society.

Centering race as a focal point of leadership development, MPLI offers a counter-narrative to the widely held standard of white leadership by orienting participants to expertise and experiences from Black and Brown leaders and communities. Integrating social contexts in leadership development is a meaningful way to leverage a community's strengths and build overall capacity (Galloway, 1997). It also helps shift the focal point from the individual to processes and practices that make race evident (Ospina, 2017). Participants witnessed firsthand their own ability to engage in leadership practices and witnessed the leadership of communities of color largely absent from the dominant political narrative. Experiential engagement with community members created opportunities for the emergence of self and the group around racial equity.

Leader and leadership development must be emphasized together as part of a broader community narrative (Porr, 2011). Shifting the program's content from solely individual political aspirations to supporting collective aspirations was an effective strategy for deploying equity-minded leaders into their communities of practice. Understanding leadership from the community standpoint is critical for a meaningfully rich leadership development experience. Exposure to local leaders of color transforms participants' and community members' experiential learning into lived expertise. Connecting the community's voice to the program helped participants translate the standpoint of these lived experiences back into their work.

MPLI underscored the requirement for complete structural change and solutions through participation in racial equity analysis. A structural view of race helped participants analyze and challenge dominant theories of practice that intersect to produce racialized outcomes (Bonilla-Silva, 1997). MPLI achieved this by implementing an intensive, team project-based learning experience designed to analyze racial equity in legislation. There is recognizable strength in uniting individuals in collective solutions to social problems (Checkoway, 1997). By deliberately focusing on racial equity in a community setting, participants could retain their focus on community goals rather than self-centered aspirations. Participants build skills to center a race-conscious approach in their leadership development by assessing and evaluating information with a critical framework (Pulliam, 2017). This informs their ability to challenge and advocate for better policy outcomes.

Conclusion

MPLI was reported to positively impact participants' understanding and ability to address racial inequity and create "racial equity prepared" leaders. The integration of CRT and leadership development helped leaders appraise their professional practice in the broader social justice movement against a narrative that has largely excluded anyone not white (Brown, 2009). Following the program, participants perceived their personal success and community outcomes to be inextricably linked. Findings also suggested the perceived increase in self-efficacy would lead to greater collective efficacy. MPLI further substantiates the personal is political. It demonstrates the ability to engage leaders across broad racial equity experiences and is uniquely situated for use as a best practice model to connect individual and collective leadership.

Acknowledgments

We would like to thank the MPLI participants, members of the Virginia Legislative Black Caucus and the many community members, scholars, and leaders for their willingness to share their time and expertise with MPLI and the researchers.

Disclosure statement

No potential conflict of interest was reported by the author(s).

ORCID

Nakeina E. Douglas-Glenn ⓘ http://orcid.org/0000-0001-8567-1513

References

Azzam, T., & Riggio, R. E. (2003). Community based leadership programs: A descriptive investigation. *Journal of Leadership and Organizational Studies*, 10(1), 55–67. https://doi.org/10.1177/2F107179190301000105

Bandura, A. (1997). *Self-efficacy: The exercise of control*. W. H. Freeman.

Bonilla-Silva, E. (1997). Rethinking racism: Toward a structural interpretation. *American Sociological Review*, 62(3), 465–480. https://doi.org/10.2307/2657316

Bono, J. E., Shen, W., & Snyder, M. (2010). Fostering integrative community leadership. *The Leadership Quarterly*, 21(2), 324–335. https://dx.doi.org/10.1016/j.leaqua.2010.01.010

Brown, N. L. (2009). Fusing Critical Race Theory with practice to improve mentorship. *International Forum of Teaching and Studies*, 5(2), 18–21.

Carton, A. M., & Rosette, A. S. (2011). Explaining bias against black leaders: Integrating theory on information processing and goal-based stereotyping. *Academy of Management Journal*, 54(6), 1141–1158. https://doi.org/10.5465/amj.2009.0745

Chandler, J. L. S., & Kirsch, R. E. (2018). Address race and culture within a critical leadership approach. In J. L. Chin, J. E. Trimble, & J. E. Garcia (Eds.), *Global and culturally diverse leaders and leadership: New dimensions and challenges for business, education and society* (pp. 307–321). Emerald Publishing.

Checkoway, B. (1997). Core concepts for community change. *Journal of Community Practice*, 4 (1), 11–29. https://doi.org/10.1300/J125v04n01_02

Christian, M., Louise, S., & Ray, V. (2019). New directions in Critical Race Theory and sociology: Racism, white supremacy, and resistance: PROD. *The American Behavioral Scientist*, 63(13), 1731–1740. https://doi.org/10.1177/0002764219842623

Constable, G., (Host). (2021, February 25). *The Westham Project: A look at Freeman* [Audio podcast episode]. In *The Collegian UR beneath the surface*. University of Richmond. https://www.thecollegianur.com/article/2021/02/the-westham-project-a-look-at-freeman

Creswell, J. W., & Creswell, J. D. (2017). *Research design: Qualitative, quantitative, and mixed methods approaches*. SAGE Publications.

Curral, L., Marques-Quinteiro, P., Gomes, C., & Lind, P. G. (2016). Leadership as an emergent feature in social organizations: Insights from a laboratory simulation experiment. *PloS One*, 11(12), e0166697. https://doi.org/10.1371/journal.pone.0166697

Day, D. V., & Harrison, M. M. (2007). A multilevel, identity-based approach to leadership development. *Human Resource Management Review*, 17(4), 360–373. https://doi.org/10.1016/j.hrmr.2007.08.007

Delgado, R., Stefancic, J., & Harris, A. (2001). *Critical Race Theory: An introduction.* NYU Press.

Dudziak, S., & Profitt, N. J. (2012). Group work and social justice: Designing pedagogy for social change. *Social Work with Groups*, 35(3), 235–252. https://doi.org/10.1080/01609513.2011.624370

Dugan, J. P. (2017). *Leadership theory: Cultivating critical perspectives.* John Wiley & Sons.

Enchautegui, M. E. (2015, May 25). *Latinos and African Americans: Shared experiences, shared solutions.* Urban wire: Race and ethnicity. https://www.urban.org/urban-wire/latinos-and-african-americans-shared-experiences-shared-solutions

Evers, C. W., & Wu, E. H. (2006). On generalising from single case studies: Epistemological reflections. *Journal of Philosophy of Education*, 40(2), 511–526. https://doi.org/10.1111/j.1467-9752.2006.00519.x

Fredericks, S. M. (1999). Exposing and exploring state-wide community leadership training programs. *Journal of Leadership and Organizational Studies*, 5(2), 129–142. https://doi.org/10.1177/2F107179199900500211

Fredericks, S. M. (2003). Creating and maintaining networks among leaders: An exploratory case study of two leadership training programs. *Journal of Leadership and Organizational Studies*, 10(1), 45–54. https://doi.org/10.1177/2F107179190301000104

Furman, G. (2012). Social justice leadership as praxis: Developing capacities through preparation programs. *Educational Administration Quarterly*, 48(2), 191–229. https://doi.org/10.1177/0013161X11427394

Galloway, R. (1997). Community leadership programs: New implications for local leadership enhancement, economic development, and benefits for regional industries. *Economic Development Review*, 15(2), 6–10. https://www.proquest.com/scholarly-journals/community-leadership-programs-new-implications/docview/230110063/se-2?accountid=14780.

Gooden, M., & Dantley, M. (2012). Centering race in a framework for leadership reparation. *Journal of Research on Leadership Education*, 7(2), 237–253. https://doi.org/10.1177/2F1942775112455266

Gurdjian, P., Halbeisen, T., & Lane, K. (2014). *Why leadership-development programs fail.* McKinsey & Company. https://www.mckinsey.com/featured-insights/leadership/why-leadership-development-programs-fail

Halkias, D., & Neubert, M. (2020). Extension of theory in leadership and management studies using the multiple-case study design. *International Leadership Journal*, 12(2), 48–73. http://internationalleadershipjournal.com/wp-content/uploads/2020/05/ILJ_Summer2020.pdf

Hannah, S. T., Avolio, B. J., Luthans, F., & Harms, P. D. (2008). Leadership efficacy: Review and future directions. *The Leadership Quarterly*, 19(6), 669–692. https://doi.org/10.1016/j.leaqua.2008.09.007

Haynie, K. (2002). The color of their skin or the content of their behavior? Race and perceptions of African American legislators. *Legislative Studies Quarterly*, 27(2), 295–314. https://doi.org/10.2307/3598532

Khine, K. (2019). *Diversity among Asians in Virginia.* Stat Chat. https://statchatva.org/2019/01/11/diversity-among-asians-in-virginia/

Murphy, S. E., & Ensher, E. A. (1999). The effects of leader and subordinate characteristics in the development of leader–member exchange quality. *Journal of Applied Social Psychology*, 29(7), 1371–1394. https://doi.org/10.1111/j.1559-1816.1999.tb00144.x

Ospina, S. M. (2017). Collective leadership and context in public administration: Bridging public leadership research and leadership studies. *Public Administration Review*, 77(2), 275–287. https://doi.org/10.1111/puar.12706

Ospina, S., & Foldy, E. (2009). A critical review of race and ethnicity in the leadership literature: Surfacing context, power and the collective dimensions of leadership. *The Leadership Quarterly*, 20(6), 876–896. https://doi.org/10.1016/j.leaqua.2009.09.005

Paglis, L. L., & Green, S. G. (2002). Leadership self-efficacy and managers' motivation for leading change. *Journal of Organizational Behavior*, 23(2), 215–235. https://doi.org/10.1002/job.137

Patton, M. Q. (2015). *Qualitative research & evaluation methods: Integrating theory and practice* (4th ed.). SAGE Publications.

Porr, D. A. (2011). Putting "development" back into community leadership (development) programs. *Community Development*, 42(1), 97–105. https://doi.org/10.1080/15575330.2010.505295

powell, j. a. (2013). Deepening our understanding of structural marginalization. *Poverty & Race*, 22(5), 3–13. http://www.prrac.org/newsletters/sepoct2013.pdf.

Pulliam, R. M. (2017). Practical application of Critical Race Theory: A social justice course design. *Journal of Social Work Education*, 53(3), 414–423. https://doi.org/10.1080/10437797.2016.1275896

Rosette, A. S., Leonardelli, G. J., & Phillips, K. W. (2008). The white standard: Racial bias in leader categorization. *Journal of Applied Psychology*, 93(4), 758. https://doi.org/10.1037/0021-9010.93.4.758

Saito, L. T. (2009). *The politics of exclusion: The failure of race-neutral policies in urban America*. Stanford University Press.

Smith, J. D. (2002). *Managing white supremacy: Race, politics, and citizenship in Jim Crow Virginia*. University of North Carolina Press.

Stech, E. (2008). Leadership education, training, and development. *Journal of Leadership Education*, 7(1), 43–46. https://doi.org/10.12806/V7/I1/C1

Thomas, J. (2019). *The Virginia way: Democracy and power after 2016*. The History Press.

Valdes, G. A. (2001). *The role of community leadership programs in fostering diversity*. (Order No. 3031443) (ProQuest Dissertations Publishing) [Doctoral Dissertation, Arizona State University]. ProQuest Dissertations & Theses Global. https://www.proquest.com/docview/251717438?accountid=14780

Van De Valk, L. J. (2008). Leadership development and social capital: Is there a relationship? *Journal of Leadership Education*, 7(1), 47–64. https://doi.org/10.12806/V7/I1/C2

Waite, S. R. (2021). Disrupting dysconsciousness: Confronting anti-Blackness in educational leadership preparation programs. *Journal of School Leadership*, 31(1–2), 66–84. https://doi.org/10.1177/1052684621993047

Weng, S. S., & Clark, P. G. (2017). In pursuit of social justice: Emic and etic perspectives of social service providers. *Journal of Community Practice*, 25(3–4), 287–308. https://doi.org/10.1080/10705422.2017.1347118

Wilson, P. (2017, February 18). *Some hope to increase diversity among Virginia legislative aides*. Richmond Times-Dispatch. https://richmond.com/news/local/government-politics/some-hope-to-increase-diversity-among-va-legislative-aides/article_a2a19610-270e-5897-b9bc-316704dc00d5.html

Yin, R. K. (2018). *Case study research and applications: Design and methods*. SAGE Publications.

Toward authentic university-community engagement

Mark G. Chupp ⓘ, Adrianne M. Fletcher, and James P. Graulty ⓘ

ABSTRACT

University-community engagement (UCE) tends to be unequal, yielding greater benefits to the university. This creates mistrust, particularly between the university and African American neighborhoods. We propose a model of authentic UCE that builds reciprocity and trust between members of the community and university and increases their capacity to collaboratively problem solve. Through experiential learning, participants confront implicit biases, and develop empathy and stamina to confront systemic racism. Through five training workshops and action circles, participants developed strategies for using their learning to address real-life issues. Lessons learned from this model might be instructive for other universities seeking more authentic UCE.

Urban universities have a troubled history with their surrounding neighborhoods (Keith, 2015; White, 2008). Related research has traditionally focused on the agenda of the researcher, not on the needs and interests of the community (Nye & Schramm, 1999; White, 2008). The very nature of the university campus as a self-contained community further exacerbates alienation from the community-at-large. Over time, universities have heeded the criticism and sought to alter the nature of their research in communities from seeing residents as simply research subjects to engaging in research that serves the public good (Boyer, 1996).

Beyond research, the relationships between universities and the surrounding communities are multifaceted and complex. While universities contribute economically, and bring an influx of human capital, they also compete for land, create artificial barriers to inclusion, and use their resources in ways that result in harmful power imbalances (Clifford & Petrescu, 2012). In the 1990s, universities actively pursued mutually beneficial community engagement and the development of university-community partnerships (Bruning et al., 2006; Fitzgerald et al., 2021).

University-community engagement (UCE) has become a major focus in higher education. Commonly held goals are to exchange knowledge, foster mutuality, create reciprocity, and contribute to the public good (Mtawa &

Wangenge-Ouma, 2021). This study examines one model of UCE – Foundations of Community Building (FCB) – an innovative community building program, which we initiated at the Community Innovation Network, a community practice center within the School of Social Work at Case Western Reserve University (a private university in Cleveland, Ohio). We founded this 8-month, non-academic learning experience to build capacity, foster mutually trusting relationships, and serve as the foundation for transforming the relationship between the university and the predominantly Black neighborhoods that surround it. This paper examines the format and lessons from one model of UCE as a demonstration of how to narrow the social distance between a university and historically oppressed neighborhoods. What we learned can be instructive for others wanting to move toward more authentic UCE.

In this paper, we first examine the history, roles, and challenges of UCE for institutions and communities. Subsequently, we describe our case study, including FCB's context and structure. Following a brief discussion of our methods, we offer an in-depth perspective on FCB, including survey, network analysis, and post-program interview results to demonstrate how this program offers new insights into UCE.

Overview of university-community engagement

In response to criticism of the university as an ivory tower, Boyer's (1996) groundbreaking work introduced a lens for the scholarship of engagement. Boyer promoted the notion of higher education advancing the public good, specifically as a "partner in the search for answers to our most pressing social, civic, economic, and moral problems." (p. 18). A few years later, with a focus on land grant and public universities, the Kellogg Commission found in its 1999 report that universities had become unresponsive to the very communities they were intended to serve. The Commission advocated that an engaged institution must "put its critical resources (knowledge and expertise) to work on the problems the communities it serves face" (Kellogg Commission on the Future of State and Land-Grant Universities, 1999, p. 10). Beginning in 1970, the Carnegie Commission on Higher Education established a framework for assessing institutions' relationships to the community and to public good. In 2005, they added the Carnegie Community Engagement Classification, a self-assessment accreditation for which institutions voluntarily apply (Public Purpose Institute, n.d.). This process provides a rigorous framework for operationalizing UCE.

According to the Carnegie Foundation for the Advancement of Teaching, community engagement is defined as "collaboration between institutions of higher education and their larger communities (local, regional/state, national, global) for the mutually beneficial exchange of knowledge and resources in a context of partnership and reciprocity" (D. J. Weerts & Sandmann, 2008, p. 74). While there is broad consensus on this definition, the specific constructs of UCE can include many things. Olson and Brennan (2017) identified common engagement themes: embodying and promoting democracy; fostering partnerships of shared power, resources and knowledge among universities, communities, and the public/private sectors; and social impact.

Over time, the community engagement framework has replaced earlier conceptualizations of service, outreach, extension, community development and community-based education. The focus is increasingly on UCE and partnerships characterized by mutually beneficial processes that lead to knowledge creation and exchange between the university and community (Mtawa et al., 2016). According to D. Weerts and Sandmann (2010), engagement should emphasize a two-way approach of collaboration between institutions and communities that aims to (1) address/acknowledge specific, relevant needs; and (2) emphasize strengths and assets in the community.

For authentic UCE, a university needs to establish reciprocity in learning and engagement that creates a flow between the institution and the residents. Saltmarsh and Zlotkowski (2011) write that reciprocity should be "inclusive, collaborative, and problem-oriented work, in which academics share knowledge-generating tasks with the public and involve community partners as participants in public problem solving" (p. 272). We propose, then, that for university-community engagement to be authentic, it requires two-way knowledge exchange; mutually beneficial relationships; reciprocity; and collaborative work on relevant problems or goals identified by the community itself. Given the historic unequal relationships and power dynamics, university-community engagement must also integrate a racial equity lens and a commitment to confront inherent power differentials.

University-community relationships are typically lopsided and yield greater benefits to the university. While the construct of UCE offers goals for a more equitable and inclusive approach, it does not provide methods for achieving these salient goals. We sought to create a capacity-building program that recognizes historic mistrust and intentionally seeks to build reciprocity, mutuality, and trust between members of the community and the university.

The outcomes of the program might serve as the foundation for a change in the narrative about the relationship and lead the institution to shift its commitments, policies and practices to align with equity and inclusion. This study addresses how to operationalize a commitment to UCE that achieves these key elements. This work is designed as a community building effort, defined as "the process of strengthening the ability of neighborhood residents, organizations, and institutions to foster and sustain neighborhood change, both individually and collectively" (Kubisch et al., 2002, p. 26).

This study seeks to answer two questions: *How effective was Foundations of Community Building in: (1) building reciprocity, mutuality, and trust between members of the community and the university, where mistrust has occurred in the past; and (2) increasing the capacity of individuals in the community and the university to be able to collaborate together on problems relevant to the community?*

A case study in university community engagement

In many urban settings, universities are resource-rich, racially whiter than the adjoining community, and often islanded physically and psychologically from the surrounding community. Urban universities historically tower over adjoining Black communities with visible and invisible doors that serve as checkpoints to keep out neighborhood members, and to keep in the university's students, faculty and staff. According to Harris (2015), exclusionary practices are not surprising as American universities have a long history with racism – including the slave trade, slavery itself, and the use of slave labor to build physical institutions.

Case Western Reserve University (CWRU), located on Cleveland, Ohio's historically Black east side, is no exception. In 2020, of CWRU's 11,500 undergraduate students, 52% identified as white and only 6% identified as Black or African American – in a city that is 49% Black. As in many cities, neighborhoods that identify as Black sit in the shadow of the university and find themselves replete with historical and current trauma in the form of severe economic challenges, poverty, deteriorating homes, crime, and university encroachment for expansion purposes (Baldwin, 2017; Ehlenz, 2015; Semuels, 2015). Structural and systemic anti-Black racism covertly drives ideologies that inform policies and practices that thwart business growth and development in these communities. This helps explain the largely missing amicable university engagement in neighborhoods that surround the university.

Confronting racism and disparities requires shifting power, reframing narratives and cultivating equitable partnerships. Building equitable partnerships is not possible without building trust between the partners, a process that begins with individual relationships. We are faculty and staff at the Jack, Joseph and Morton Mandel School of Applied Social Sciences (social work) at CWRU. In general, schools of social work are well positioned to lead this change and our school has a history of community practice and community engaged scholarship. We are affiliated with the Community Innovation Network, a center that seeks to increase community trust and narrow the social distance between the university and community.

Foundations of Community Building (FCB) is a program we designed to purposefully build capacity, mutual trust, and collaborative within-cohort problem-solving via a comprehensive five-part strength-based curriculum and an experiential learning process. The FCB curriculum focuses on transformative approaches at the individual, interpersonal, community, and system levels. Five capacity-building training sessions over eight months are infused with a racial equity lens. The first training session, Change Agents Unite, focuses on empowerment of each person as a change agent (organizer, facilitator) in their community or organization. The next two training sessions focus on Asset Based Community Development (ABCD) and Appreciative Inquiry (AI), strength-based strategies for building community change by leveraging existing assets. The last two training sessions focus on inclusive facilitation skills and conflict transformation, providing participants the methods and skills for building bridges across differences and uniting people for a cause. All training sessions are co-led by a diverse training team. Case studies and exercises are drawn from communities encountering similar dynamics.

Recruitment methods are intentional. We considered the roles of historical trauma and racism on Black persons who reside within the adjoining, high-poverty neighborhoods. The program includes a cohort comprised of 50% neighborhood residents and representatives from community-based organizations (CBOs) and 50% representatives from the university.[1] Recruiting a diverse and representative cohort is essential. The university provost provided scholarships to cover fees for residents, along with a $1,500 stipend (increased to $2,000 for Cohort 2). Cohort 1 took place between October 2018 and June 2019 and included 11 residents from three adjoining neighborhoods, and 12 institutional members (9 from the university and 3 from other institutions in University Circle). In this cohort, 15 participants were Black or Latinx, and eight were white. The Chief of University Circle Police, the community relations director for the CWRU Police, a director of a medical school research center, and the director of the university's office of local government and community relations participated.

The second cohort took place from January to September 2020, interrupted by the COVID-19 pandemic with a three-month hiatus and included seven residents from five adjoining neighborhoods, six from community-based organizations, 10 participants from the university and one from the nearby Cleveland Clinic. In this cohort, 13 participants were Black, nine were white, two were other. Strong university representation continued in Cohort 2, which included a social work faculty member and the university's new associate provost for interprofessional education, research and collaborative practice.

FCB is an experiential learning process. In the first retreat-like session, participants interact around their passions and values without disclosing their professional status, titles, or levels of education. Getting to know the person for who they are precedes knowing about their affiliations. Another

Leveling the Engagement Field
1. Name tags with first names without formal position designation.
2. The breaking of bread at each event with catering from local, minority-owned businesses
3. Land Acknowledgement: This Indigenous practice acknowledges historic harm
4. The Wall Activity: Participants place sticky-notes My Time/My Self Care and Group Norms
5. Paired Conversations (Participants sit knee-to-knee and share a memory of their community).
6. Movement Moments: Short choreographed activities allow participants to bring their entire selves into the space by way of rhythmical active movement).
7. Knee-to-Knee Conversations in Threes: Participants respond to the following questions: (1) What is a commitment you hold that brought you into this room today? (2) How valuable an experience do you plan to have in this space? (3) What is a gift that you are afraid of using? (Block, 2009).
8. The Looking Glass Self Exercise: Participants share with one other person who they believe the other person thinks them to be and why, revealing hidden biases (Crawford Fletcher, 2019).

Figure 1. Leveling the engagement field.

important experience which takes place during the first FCB session is The Looking Glass Self, which raises awareness of one's own implicit or unconscious bias. According to Marsh (2009) implicit biases, either positive or negative function outside of our awareness. The components of implicit bias – prejudice, discrimination and stereotyping – are part and parcel of every human (Marsh, 2009). Unless these factors are brought into one's awareness, they will bring damage to themselves and others. Mitigating the deleterious influence of race, racism, and anti-Black racism within FCB occurs during the first two days by intentionally breaking down barriers, leveling the playing field, and establishing caring personal relationships that promote trust across differences. See Figure 1.

Throughout the 8-month process, participants actively engage in *Learning and Action Circles*. Facilitators led a process to surface issues of relevance that the cohort wanted to work on. Affinity groups were then formed, with a deliberate mix of neighborhood residents, representatives from CBOs, and the university/institutions.

Study aims and methods

To answer our research questions, we evaluated FCB as an experiential learning program, measuring changes in trust building, capacity building, networking, and the collective power of participants to create change. The evaluation of Cohort 1 consisted of satisfaction surveys at the end of each workshop and a final program evaluation after the fifth workshop. These surveys were developed utilizing the FCB logic model. There were 18 participants in the evaluation: six residents, five from CBOs, and seven from University Circle institutions.

Cohort 2's evaluation included the same session evaluations as Cohort 1 plus a pre- and post-survey in four key areas based on the FCB model: program organization; capacity building; community engagement/collaboration; and relationship/ trust-building. These surveys were also developed using the program logic model, and were informed by existing research (Frey et al., 2006; Leppin et al., 2018; Yamagishi & Yamagishi, 1994). Given the small sample size, we completed a descriptive analysis of the survey data.

Cohort 2 participants also completed a pre- and post-network analysis. Each participant was asked to rate on a four-point scale their level of connection, and level of trust at the beginning and end of the program (refer to Table 1 below). The item about connection is from Ehrlichman and Spence (2018); the items about trust were adapted from the work of Sampson et al. (1997). Network analysis measured the change in ratings at an individual level, person to person for each cohort member. These changes were then aggregated to draw conclusions about connection and trust within and across sectors (resident, CBOs, institution).

In total, 17 of the 24 participants in Cohort 2 responded to the post program evaluation and post network analysis: eight from the university (all white), four from CBOs in the neighborhoods (two Black, one white, one chose not to identify), and five neighborhood residents (four Black, one Multi-Racial). The pre-survey and pre-network analysis were conducted on paper immediately after the training, with 100% participation. Due to the COVID-19 pandemic, post-surveys were conducted electronically, reducing the participation rate.

In Cohort 2, 11 participants – five from institutions (three white, one Black, one Asian), three CBOs (two Black, one white), and three residents (all Black) also shared their insights in qualitative interviews conducted five months after the program ended. We asked 12 questions about their FCB experience and mutual trusting relationships; race and racism; access to institutions; perception of neighborhoods; power sharing; and collaboration. Interviews were

Table 1. Change in connections and trust between pre- and post-network analyses.

Average change in response from pre to post (max change of 3):	1. Rate your level of connection with this Person	2. Would you feel comfortable enough to have this person over to your home for a meal?	3. Would you feel comfortable enough to have a dialogue with this person about what might be a difficult topic (conflict, race relations, etc.)	4. Would you feel comfortable enough to turn to this person if you need help with a personal problem?	Average of the 3 preceding questions to approximate average change in trust
U→U	1.54	0.73	0.58	0.97	0.76
U→CBO	1.21	0.58	0.17	0.73	0.49
U→R	1.34	0.78	0.40	0.79	0.66
CBO→U	1.60	0.83	0.57	1.60	1.00
CBO→CBO	1.33	0.93	0.60	1.47	1.00
CBO→R	1.52	0.95	0.76	1.60	1.10
R→U	1.23	1.43	1.33	0.93	1.23
R→CBO	0.83	1.58	1.42	0.92	1.31
R→R	1.46	1.75	1.63	1.04	1.47

conducted via Zoom by graduate field interns and lasted between 30 and 50 minutes in length. Participants' responses were recorded, transcribed, and then categorized to identify common themes. The themes were then rated by prevalence and the intensity with which participants spoke about the theme. These scores were aggregated to determine the most salient themes.

Findings

The findings focus on the effectiveness of FCB in building the knowledge and capacity of university and neighborhood participants; developing mutually beneficial trusting relationships; and establishing a collaborative process for addressing problems or concerns relevant to the community. We will discuss the key takeaways for each focus area, based on the general findings of each instrument: (1), the Cohort 1 post-training and post-cohort survey; (2) the Cohort 2 pre- and post-session surveys; Cohort 2 final survey; and Cohort 2 pre- and post-program network analysis. Evaluations show that FCB was successful in its goals of developing relationships of mutual trust, and building knowledge and capacity among cohort members.

FCB increased all participants' knowledge and skills. In Cohort 1, 100% of participants reported that they gained new skills and resources; used and shared the materials and resources; and became knowledgeable and gained exposure to the foundational aspects of community building. In Cohort 2, 100% rated gaining knowledge of the foundational aspects of community building as good or excellent (82%). 94% rated their ability to identify challenges and create solutions with residents, CBOs and institutions as good or excellent (70%). This finding is also supported by the qualitative interviews, specifically Themes 2 and 4, as seen in Table 2 below. One resident participant reported: "(FCB) gives me a perspective to know that I live in an environment where changes can be made, and we can start something bigger than just me ... Here it shows me that we can do something big and do something different."

All groups – participants from University Circle Institutions (U), those who work for Community Based Organizations (CBO), and Residents (R) of area neighborhoods residents – increased their level of connection with each other. This increase was largest for participants who work in community-based organizations, and their relationships increased the most with all three participant groups. The chart in Table 1 shows the pre- and post-network analysis average change in response to each question in aggregate for each identity group.

This chart was created by taking each participant's post-network rating of every other participant and subtracting their pre-network rating. These scores were then grouped by identity (U, CBO, R) and then the ratings were averaged. So, Question 1, Row **CBO→U** indicates a score of 1.60. This means, on

BEYOND LIP SERVICE

Table 2. Top themes from the cohort 2 qualitative interviews.

Theme	Representative Quotes
1. The environment allowed authentic selves to show up, and created space for trust (Relationships)	"I think that especially the vibe set up by [the team], really established that it was a safe space that was welcoming." – *CBO* "People were genuine, they were listening, they were open and curious, and it was just overwhelming for me and it gave me, I guess, a feeling of safety. That I can be authentic like I could just share and I knew it would be received." – *University/Institution*
2. Increased capacity for reckoning with the legacy of systemic racism (Capacity)	"The first session really just blew me away and it got me thinking about race and the dynamics of race [...] and how much those dynamics impact community building and community development." – *CBO* "I'm not around white people all the time, [...] and to see how people feel, and what they want to do to change this or the overwhelming guilt they feel, it allowed me to see their perspective. – *Resident*
3. Most respondents have maintained connection with other participants despite the pandemic (Relationships)	"I have been emailing with a few of the community members [...] and have met by zoom, but [...] with the pandemic we're not able to do quite as much in the community." – *University/Institution* "Towards the end of the session I was starting a book club that was Community based and inspired out of the unrest of 2020. [...] One person has joined and become a regular participant." – *Resident*
4. Increased knowledge and skills for community building (Capacity)	"FCB brought [...] cohesive information and assistance in regards to the bigger picture. It gave me more and better insight, better tools, and everything else." – *Resident* "Because of these connections and learning about the makeup of the community and working with the CDCs and everything. I think it showed me what was possible." – *University/Institution*
5. Switching to virtual negatively impacted the action circle projects (Collaborative Process)	"[Doing things via Zoom] had a pretty significant impact on our project, but it didn't have an impact, I don't think as much on the actual cohesion of our group of people. – *University/Institution* "Had it been in person, some of us would have met for coffee. I'm more of a person-to-person person. I think the virtual nature of it was great in some ways, while in other ways, it prevented intimacy because, you just don't want to be on Zoom that much." – *CBO*
6. FCB connected participants, and broke down barriers between groups (Relationships)	"One thing that I liked was not differentiating who is a resident, who is an institutional person, etc. I think that allows for everyone to be in the space and not perform their titles, and allows them to bring their full self to this work that we're doing together." – *CBO* "I think everybody was pretty open to learning and open to new ideas." – *Resident*
7. Improved mutuality of relationships (Relationships)	"I made the connections with people from these institutions, so if I wanted to do something or get us to all work together on a project, I know the people that I need to contact in order to make stuff happen." – *Resident* "I think that it's recognizing that people in the community, if you're doing something for them, they should have a voice at the table." -*University/Institution*

average, CBO members rated their level of connectedness with U members, 1.60 points higher on the post-survey than on the pre-survey. A rating less than 0 would indicate a decrease in connection or trust. Any rating between 0 and 0.75 means that on average, there was a small increase, between 0.75 and 1.5 would be a significant increase, and anything above 1.5 is a large increase from pre- to post-survey.

All participants reported a growth in their trusting relationships through the program. In Cohort 1, 100% of respondents reported that they built trusting relationships with participants who were residents and from community-based organizations through the program. Almost all (95%) reported that they built trusting relationships with institution representatives. Two-thirds of all participants reported increased participation in community events. In Cohort 2, 94% responded with good or excellent (88%) to the item, "Participants of diverse cultures and backgrounds are respected, heard, and valued in this cohort."

For the second cohort, we added measures on how trust increased. In the Cohort 2 network analysis, many participants gave high ratings in the pre-network analysis for sharing a meal at home and for engaging in dialogue on a difficult topic. The average response for the meal question was 2.18 and 2.55 for the dialogue question. This is compared to average responses of 1.32 for the personal problem question and an average of 1.18 for the connection ratings. These pre-program findings indicate that the cohort consisted of people who are naturally more trusting than the general population. This is important to consider when interpreting Table 1, because a higher baseline lowers the possible average increase that we can observe from pre- to post-measurement, and increases the possibility of a negative result.

Despite the high baselines for the questions on trust, we still observed a significant increase in trust between the three groups as seen in Table 1. On average, residents' trust of participants from the University, CBOs, and each other, rose the most out of the three groups. One contributing factor is that residents' ratings on the first two items were lower on average than the other two groups on the pre-network analysis, so they had the most room for change from baseline. By the post-network analysis, residents' responses were in line with the average responses of other groups, indicating that residents had started the program with lower levels of trust, but that trust had risen to comparable levels through the program. In short, through this eight-month program, residents built trusting relationships with others. These findings are also supported by Themes 1, 3, 6, and 7 from the qualitative interviews, shown in Table 2.

Through qualitative interviews, we learned what specifically contributed to the increase in knowledge and skills and to more trusting relationships. Five months after the conclusion of Cohort 2, we conducted qualitative interviews. The key themes that emerged are listed in rank order in Table 2, along with quotes from participants that speak to each theme. Almost all participants reported that the program strengthened their ability to address problems. In Cohort 1, 100% of participants reported that they identified challenges and concrete solutions toward increased community engagement. 87% reported good or higher on the helpfulness of learning circles in applying content. In Cohort 2, participants identified their Top 3 community building challenges in the pre-survey. In the post, more than 94% reported their ability to respond to these challenges as good or excellent. One resident said: "We plan to continue meeting as a group virtually because we feel strongly about saving our community."

One Action Circle from Cohort 1 continued to meet and developed a proposal for the establishment of a permanent university-affiliated Neighborhood Advisory Council. CWRU approved the charter, which makes racial equity an explicit goal and stipulates that residents – who receive compensation for their participation – make up the majority of the Council.

While we set out to strengthen the role of the Action Circles in cohort 2, one challenge was the interruption of the COVID-19 pandemic, which emerged halfway through the program. Cohort 2 participants spoke about this in the qualitative interviews, particularly in Theme 5 (see Table 2). We did not realize the anticipated highly engaged, self-organizing Action Circles to address the major challenges they had identified at the start of the program.

Conclusions and lessons learned

The findings suggest that FCB is effective at cultivating trusting relationships across diverse participants from the community and university. Participants gained knowledge and skills in approaches for promoting change, although this did not generally result in concrete outcomes. While results were positive for Cohort 2, the pandemic hampered the ability to foster deeper relationships and work collaboratively together. In future cohorts, we will include more robust pre- and post-surveys to fully measure self- and collective efficacy (Ohmer, 2007). This, and more rigorous and relevant Learning and Action Circles, will provide clearer measurable short-term outcomes of the program.

Overall, there are several lessons learned that others considering initiating programs like FCB as a means to more authentic UCE might benefit from:

(1) To ensure that UCE leads to authentic collaborative problem solving, a more intentional development of the action teams is needed. Trusting relationships provide a good basis for identifying and working on relevant issues and change goals. Recruiting participants into the cohort based on a commitment to work on specific issues might be helpful.

(2) Building equity between neighborhoods and the university requires greater participation over time and integration into institutional change efforts. FCB used our resources to level the playing field versus further-ing the historic power imbalance (Clifford & Petrescu, 2012) by assuring that 50% of FCB's recruits were community members. Minority-owned

businesses and vendors from the neighborhoods were also hired to support the FCB trainings. Institutionalizing FCB and integrating it into a university's strategic plan is one way to promote change. Uniting previous cohorts around a shared agenda would also affect positive change.

(3) The process of intentional participant narrative sharing within small group settings elevates the common humanity of diverse participants. This process brings to the forefront the collective participant experience and leads to a refreshing, bi-directional dissemination of expertise and knowledge, exemplifying the public good as proposed by Mtawa and Wangenge-Ouma (2021). The bi-directional dissemination of expertise and knowledge raises awareness of the creative and entrepreneurial strengths and assets of the community and specific community members, which were then magnified by the skills, talents and abilities of university scholars. This activity supports Weerts and Sandmann (2010) notion of two-way collaboration.

(4) Building capacity and trusting relationships will not alone shift power. However, a program like FCB can provide the foundation of trusting relationships for building more equitable partnerships. We also recommend linking FCB to larger investments in structural change, such as the Community Engagement Centers and long-term commitment to neighborhoods at the University of Pittsburgh (University of Pittsburgh, 2019).

(5) Programs like FCB should be linked to the strengthening or development of longer-term partnerships. FCB worked toward building partnerships by way of the creation of action teams. Intentionally organizing these into partnership provides a framework for effective community engagement as defined by the Carnegie Foundation (Public Purpose Institute, n.d.).

(6) Move away from conceptualizing the university and the community as monolithic entities. Dempsey (2010) argues that treating the community as one inappropriately assumes residents are representative or can speak on behalf of the community. Likewise, by treating the university as a self-contained unit, it minimizes the reality that some, if not many people claim their identity in both the university and community. Focusing on UCE itself reinforces these differences rather than cultivating a shared identity and common set of interests and goals.

In conclusion, there is no guarantee that the good will and capacity created in programs like FCB will lead to larger changes. White (2008) warns that "The scales of power are tilted too much in favor of the university to presume that respectful relationships with community leaders are enough to lure them into productive partnerships" (p. 133). This work is the first step; uniting together to confront power dynamics and take action to change systems must follow.

Note

1. The university subgroup included some representatives from other institutions in University Circle, a compact area comprised of CWRU and other educational, medical and cultural institutions.

Acknowledgments

We are grateful for the assistance of graduate student, Sarah Wolf who served as research assistant throughout the study and Community Innovation Network Program Coordinator, Xinyuan Cui, who assisted in program design and the evaluation process.

Disclosure statement

No potential conflict of interest was reported by the author(s).

ORCID

Mark G. Chupp (iD) http://orcid.org/0000-0003-0367-0520
James P. Graulty (iD) http://orcid.org/0000-0001-9950-6957

References

Baldwin, D. L. (2017, July 30). When universities swallow cities. *The Chronicle of Higher Education*. https://www.chronicle.com/article/when-universities-swallow-cities/

Block, P. (2009). *Community: The structure of belonging*. Berrett-Koehler Publishers.

Boyer, E. (1996). The scholarship of engagement. *Bulletin of the American Academy of Arts and Sciences, 49*(7), 18–33. https://doi.org/10.2307/3824459

Bruning, S. D., McGrew, S., & Cooper, M. (2006). Town–gown relationships: Exploring university–community engagement from the perspective of community members. *Public Relations Review, 32*(2), 125–130. https://doi.org/10.1016/j.pubrev.2006.02.005

Clifford, D., & Petrescu, C. (2012). The keys to university–community engagement sustainability. *Nonprofit Management and Leadership, 23*(1), 77–91. https://doi.org/10.1002/nml.21051

Dempsey, S. E. (2010). Critiquing community engagement. *Management Communication Quarterly, 24*(3), 359–390. https://doi.org/10.1177/0893318909352247

Ehlenz, M. M. (2015). *Anchoring communities: The impact of university interventions on neighborhood revitalization* (Publicly Accessible Penn Dissertations, 1050. https://repository.upenn.edu/edissertations/1050/

Ehrlichman, D., & Spence, M. (2018, March 15). *Asking the right questions: Collecting meaningful data about your network*. Medium. https://blog.kumu.io/asking-the-right-questions-collecting-meaningful-data-about-your-network-dcb4b5f9383c

Fitzgerald, H. E., Allen, A., & Roberts, P. (2021). Campus-community partnerships: Perspectives on engaged research. In H. E. Fitzgerald, C. Burack, & S. D. Seifer (Eds.), *Handbook of engaged scholarship* (pp. 5–28). Michigan State University. https://www.jstor.org/stable/10.14321/j.ctt7zt9br

Frey, B. B., Lohmeier, J. H., Lee, S. W., & Tollefson, N. (2006). Measuring collaboration among grant partners. *American Journal of Evaluation, 27*(3), 383–392. https://doi.org/10.1177/1098214006290356

Harris, L. M. (2015). The long, ugly history of racism at American universities. *The New Republic.* https://newrepublic.com/article/121382/forgotten-racist-past-American-universities

Keith, N. Z. (2015). *Engaging in social partnerships: Democratic practices for campus-community partnerships.* Routledge.

Kellogg Commission on the Future of State and Land-Grant Universities. (1999). *Returning to our roots: The engaged institution.* National Association of State Universities and Land-Grant Colleges. https://www.aplu.org/library/returning-to-our-roots-the-engaged-institution/file

Kubisch, A. C., Auspos, P., Brown, P., Chakin, R., Fulbright-Anderson, K., & Hamilton, R. (2002). *Voices from the field: Reflections on comprehensive community change.* The Aspen Institute. https://www.aspeninstitute.org/wp%2Dcontent/uploads/files/content/docs/rcc/voicesIIbook.pdf

Leppin, A. L., Okamoto, J. M., Organick, P. W., Thota, A. D., Barrera-Flores, F. J., Wieland, M. L., McCoy, R. G., Bonacci, R. P., & Montori, V. M. (2018). Applying social network analysis to evaluate implementation of a multisector population health collaborative that uses a bridging hub organization. *Frontiers in Public Health, 6*, 315. https://doi.org/10.3389/fpubh.2018.00315

Marsh, S. C. (2009). The lens of implicit bias. *Juvenile and Family Justice Today,* 16–19. https://judicialengagementnetwork.org/images/documents/resources/cultural_awareness/ImplicitBias.pdf

Mtawa, N. N., Fongwa, S. N., & Wangenge-Ouma, G. (2016). The scholarship of university-community engagement: Interrogating Boyer's model. *International Journal of Educational Development, 49*, 126–133. https://doi.org/10.1016/j.ijedudev.2016.01.007

Mtawa, N. N., & Wangenge-Ouma, G. (2021). Questioning private good driven university-community engagement: A Tanzanian case study. *Higher Education,* 1–15. https://doi.org/10.1007/s10734-021-00685-9

Nye, N., & Schramm, R. (1999). *Building higher education-community development corporation partnerships.* U.S. Department of Housing and Urban Development. https://community-wealth.org/sites/clone.community-wealth.org/files/downloads/tool-HUD-CED-and-univ.pdf

Ohmer, M. L. (2007). Citizen participation in neighborhood organizations and its relationship to volunteers' self- and collective efficacy and sense of community. *Social Work Research, 31*(2), 109–120. https://doi.org/10.1093/swr/31.2.109

Olson, B., & Brennan, M. (2017). From community engagement to community emergence: The holistic program design approach. *The International Journal of Research on Service-Learning and Community Engagement, 5*(1), 5–19. https://journals.sfu.ca/iarslce/index.php/journal/article/view/215

Public Purpose Institute. (n.d.). *Resources from 2015 cycle and earlier.* https://public-purpose.org/initiatives/carnegie-elective-classifications/community-engagement-classification-u-s/resources-from-2015-cycle-and-earlier/

Saltmarsh, J., & Zlotkowski, E. (2011). Characteristics of an engaged department: Design and assessment. In Saltmarsh, J., and Zlotkowski, E. (Eds.) *Higher education and democracy: Essays on service-learning and civic engagement* (pp. 266–280). Temple University Press. Retrieved July 20, 2021, from http://www.jstor.org/stable/j.ctt14bt5qz.26

Sampson, R. J., Raudenbush, S. W., & Earls, F. (1997). Neighborhoods and violent crime: A multilevel study of collective efficacy. *Science*, 277(5328), 918–924. https://doi.org/10.1126/science.277.5328.918

Semuels, A. (2015). Should urban universities help their neighbors. *The Atlantic*. https://www.theatlantic.com/business/archive/2015/01/should-urban-universities-help-their-neighbors/384614/

University of Pittsburgh. (2019, November 5). University of Pittsburgh community engagement center [Video]. *YouTube*. https://www.youtube.com/watch?v=0wp3jqJY85Y

Weerts, D. J., & Sandmann, L. R. (2008). Building a two-way street: Challenges and opportunities for community engagement at research universities. *The Review of Higher Education*, 32(1), 73–106. https://doi.org/10.1353/rhe.0.0027

Weerts, D., & Sandmann, L. (2010). Community engagement and boundary-spanning roles at research universities. *The Journal of Higher Education*, 81(6), 632–657. https://doi.org/10.1080/00221546.2010.11779075

White, B. P. (2008). *Bridging the high street divide: Community power and the pursuit of democratic partnerships between Ohio State University and Weinland Park. (2008)* (Dissertations available from ProQuest. AAI3311543). https://repository.upenn.edu/dissertations/AAI3311543

Yamagishi, T., & Yamagishi, M. (1994). Trust and commitment in the United States and Japan. *Motivation and Emotion*, 18(2), 129–166. https://doi.org/10.1007/BF02249397

Index

Abrams, L. S. 16, 20
affordable housing 73–74, 76, 78, 80, 82, 85–86
agencies 7, 29–30
Albina district 77, 79–82, 84–85
Allen-Meares, P. 13, 16, 17
Allport, G. 59, 67
anti-racist social work 18–19
anti-racist work 58, 91
Anti-Riot Act 38
awareness 95, 107, 113

backlash politics 2–9
Black people 15, 63, 66–67, 81, 84, 93
bonds, building 49–51
Bonilla-Silva, E. 12, 13
Bono, J. E. 96
Boyer, E. 103
Brennan, M. 104
Brown, W. 5
Burman, S. 13, 16

Carter, D. C. 39
CASA 45, 50–52, 54–55
Cherry, L. 19
civic participation 75–76, 82
civil disobedience 3–5
civil rights legislation 2, 5
civil rights policies 4–7
civil rights reforms 3–5
Cloward, R. A. 8
Cohen, Nathan E. 26, 27, 39
cohesion 46, 53–54, 75, 84–85
color 14–15, 21, 34, 42, 44, 64, 72–75, 86–87, 92, 95, 97–98
communities 7–9, 15–21, 28–30, 42–44, 46–49, 53, 64, 73, 75–78, 81–83, 87, 91–94, 96–98, 102–106, 112–113; building 62–64, 67, 86, 103, 105–106, 109; capacity 53; of color 15, 21, 42, 72–73, 75, 86–87, 95, 97; development programs 44–45; practice 7, 21, 97, 105; preference policies 8, 73–74, 87; safety 54; well-being 73–75, 78, 81, 85–86

community based violence 58–69
community policing 42–45, 48, 55; interventions 45–46
community-based organizations (CBOs) 43, 46, 55, 106–109, 111
community-police relations 46, 51
conservatives 34–35
Corley, N. A. 18
Cramer, D. N. 13
crime 15, 43–46, 48, 50–52, 67, 105

data analysis 92
Dempsey, S. E. 113
Detlaff, A. 16, 20
displacement 72–73, 77
DuBois, W. E. B. 33

Edmonds-Cady, C. 17
Edwards, F. 14
Ehrlichman, D. 108
equity 8, 19, 75, 78, 81–83, 96, 104
Esposito, M. 14

Fekete, L. 18, 19
focus groups 46, 48, 51, 61–62, 78–79, 81, 83, 92
Foundations of Community Building (FCB) 103, 106–107, 109, 112–113

gang prevention program 46, 54
gentrification 72–77, 85, 87
Gillon 39
Graham, A. 15
gym clients 60–62

Hackworth, J. 5
Harris, L. M. 105
higher education 92, 102–103
Holosko, M. J. 17

immigrant neighborhoods 43–44
immigration reform 3–4

INDEX

inclusion 5, 20, 38, 75, 81–83, 95, 102, 104
Indigenous people 12–16, 21
inner city weightlifting (ICW) 60–62, 64–69
intergroup contact intervention 58, 60
intergroup contact theory 59, 68–69
intervention 20, 45–46, 58–60, 67
Iverson, K. 8

Jeyasingham, D. 19

Kerner Commission 26, 38–39
knowledge 5, 18, 37, 50, 90, 93, 95, 103–104, 109, 111–113

Latinx immigrant communities 42, 44, 55
Latinx immigrant neighborhoods 43–44, 55
Lavalette, M. 19
leadership 36, 44, 90–97; development 90–91, 93–94, 97–98
Lee, H. 14
legislation 33, 95, 98
Lipsky, M. 8, 26, 39
Long, L. 15
long-term residents 75–76
Los Angeles Riot Study (LARS) 25–37, 39–40

Marsh, S. C. 107
McCone Commission 26, 39
McMahon, A. 17
militants 33–37; organizations 34
minorities 3–4, 15, 84
minoritized communities 3, 13, 95
Minority Political Leadership Institute (MPLI) 90–94, 96–98; signature features 94; vision and mission 93
Morton, J. 19
Mtawa, N. N. 113

Needleman, C. E. 7
Needleman, M. L. 7
Negro groupings, polarization 33–34
Negroes 27–38; community 32–33, 37
neighborhoods 32, 42, 44–46, 48–49, 53–54, 63, 72, 74–86, 105, 108, 112–113; gentrifying 8, 73–76, 86–87; infrastructure 49, 52; residents 104, 106–107
neoliberal policies 5–7
network 45, 62–65
Newman, Z. 14, 16

Olson, B. 104
Olson, D. J. 26, 39
Ong, P. M. 39

Penketh, L. 19
Piven, F. F. 8

place attachment 75–76, 81–82, 85
police 2, 9, 13–15, 20, 30, 43–44, 46, 49–51, 53–55; brutality 14–15, 25–26, 30, 35; shootings 13–14, 25
policies 6, 8, 36, 42, 72–74, 76–80, 85–87, 92–93, 104
Portland Housing Bureau 78
preference policies 72, 74–83, 85–87
program description 60

race/racism 2–3, 8, 12–13, 15–20, 29, 31, 60, 64–65, 67–69, 72–76, 79, 81, 83–87, 90–91, 93, 94, 96–98, 105–108
racial equity 92–98, 112; analysis 95, 98; leadership 90–98
racial justice 8, 12, 17, 19, 21, 72, 86–87
Reisch, M. 8
returning residents 76, 78, 85–86
rich white people 63, 65
Rios, V. M. 13
riot 25–29, 31–32, 35–36, 38–39

Saltmarsh, J. 104
Sampson, R. J. 108
Sandmann, L. R. 104, 113
sense of safety 43, 48, 54
silent majority 2, 5–7
Smith McElveen, J. 13
social action 8, 12, 17, 19, 31
social cohesion 46, 53, 75
social connection 75, 81
social justice 6–7, 39, 60, 90, 92, 94–96; movements 3–9
social media 13–14, 51–52
social networks 42, 62–64
social work 7–8, 15–20, 26–27, 39, 68, 103, 105; education 12, 17–18; movement 19; profession 16–17, 19
social workers 2, 6–7, 12, 16–20, 26, 39, 44, 95
southern strategy 2–3, 6
Spence, M. 108
state-wide immersion 94
systemic racism 12–13, 17–20, 87
Szetela, A. 5, 7

trust 31, 46, 50, 104–105, 107–108, 110–111; building 43, 49–50, 54, 105, 107

underserved communities 95
university-community engagement (UCE) 102–114
urban neighborhoods 73

Wangenge-Ouma, G. 113
Watts 25, 27, 29–30, 32; riots 25, 27, 39; social ills in 29–31

INDEX

Weerts, D. J. 104, 113
well-being 12, 15, 73–80, 83, 85–87; improved 79, 81
Wells Barnett, I. B. 13
White, B. P. 113
white community 26, 31–32, 35–37
white people 63, 67, 84–85

white reactions 31–32
Wingfield, T. T. 17

xeno-racism 18

Young, S. M. 18

Zlotkowski, E. 104

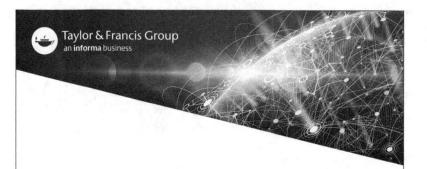

9781032415420